To our wonderful and supportive wives who are on this journey with us and who have encouraged us to write this book; and to all our children and grandchildren who will always be proud of their fathers and grandfathers for what they have done for the world.

Live to 120

A Proven Protocol for Baby Boomers

Elliot G. Levy, M.D.
Clinical Professor of Medicine (Retired)
University of Miami Miller School of Medicine
Division of Endocrinology
Miami, FL

Brian R. Clement, Ph.D., L.N.
Director, Hippocrates Wellness
West Palm Beach, FL

Table of Contents

Biographical Sketches   *vi*

Introduction   *viii*

Prologue   *xi*

CHAPTER 1   Healthy Eating   1

CHAPTER 2   Exercise   44

CHAPTER 3   Use Your Brain   60

CHAPTER 4   Socialization   66

CHAPTER 5   Spiritual Life   72

CHAPTER 6   Keep Having Sex   83

CHAPTER 7   Role of the Microbiome in Health   95

CHAPTER 8   Can Stem Cells Help?   104

CHAPTER 9   Health Care and Insurance   115

CHAPTER 10   Traditional and Complementary Medicine   124

CHAPTER 11   How and When to Retire   135

CHAPTER 12   Inflammation   141

CHAPTER 13   For the Future   149

Appendix A Going Out to Dinner   *173*

Appendix B Summary of Suggestions   *233*

Appendix C Too Good to Be True   *236*

Appendix D References   *244*

Index   *259*

Biographical Sketches

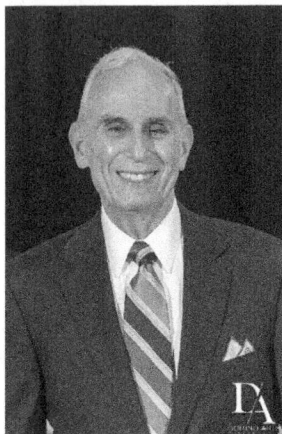

Elliot G. Levy, M.D., was born in 1946 in Kansas City, MO. He attended Carnegie-Mellon University and Northwestern University Feinberg School of Medicine, receiving his M.D. degree in 1971. He completed his residency in Internal Medicine at Washington University (St. Louis) and his fellowship in Endocrinology at the University of Southern California Keck School of Medicine. He settled in Miami, FL, in 1975 and became a Clinical Professor of Medicine at the University of Miami Miller School of Medicine, as well as having a private practice in Aventura, FL. For many years, he was known as the thought leader for thyroid problems for patients living in South Florida. He was on the Executive Council of the American Thyroid Association and was the Associate Editor of the journal, *Thyroid*. In 2005, he was honored by the Endocrine Society as the Master Clinician of the Year. He has published 38 scientific articles, authored 6 chapters in books, and has given over 300 oral presentations. His wife, Deborah Levy, Ed.D., is a nationally known authority on reading and teacher training. Together, they have three grown children and seven grandchildren. In 2001, he and his wife began their personal journey to understand what it takes to remain healthy and to apply that knowledge to their personal lives. This book is a true reflection of their beliefs. The research behind the book has provided a further impetus to doing the right things to live and enjoy life, hopefully, for 120 years.

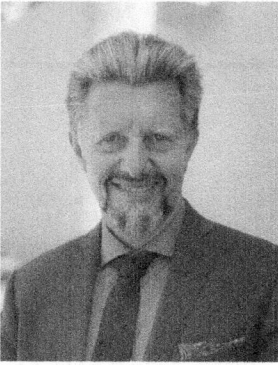

Brian R. Clement, Ph.D., L.N., was born in 1951 in New York City, NY. He has spent more than five decades researching and practicing nutrition and progressive health care. He has received graduate degrees in both naturopathic medicine and nutritional sciences. Since 1980, together with his wife, Anna Maria Clement, Ph.D., they have continued and expanded the pioneer work of Ann Wigmore and guided their Hippocrates Wellness Center (West Palm Beach, FL) into a new era that has created an expansive international acceptance of its renowned program. In his role as a health educator, Dr. Clement has conducted countless seminars, lectures, and educational programs, traveling extensively throughout the United States, as well as to more than 40 countries around the globe. In recent years, he has been commissioned by government-supported organizations to establish, organize, and direct health programs in Denmark, Ireland, Switzerland, Greece, and India. Dr. Clement's progressive ideas on natural health, coupled with his vast theoretical and practical scientific experience and his amazing teaching skills, have earned him a reputation as a leading expert in the advancing field of health. He is a great motivational speaker and has a wealth of knowledge that he constantly shares with the community. He has authored many books in the health and nutrition field including *Quantum Human, Life Force, Living Food for Optimal Health, Finding You in You, Killer Fish, Killer Clothes,* and *Dairy Deception.*

Introduction

We wrote this book for you, thriving members of the "Baby Boomer" generation, like us. We were born between 1946 and 1964. Between those years
76.4 million people had been born, representing 25% of the American population. World War II had just ended. In fact, during that first year alone, there
were 3.4 million births that occurred. Many American soldiers, called "GIs,"
had been drafted or enlisted in the U.S. Military Service. Many had been
away from home for two or even three years, often leaving a spouse at home
anxiously awaiting their return. Because of the "boom" in births that occurred
over the next 18 years, the generation was labeled as "Baby Boomers."

There is no definite answer as to what caused the baby boom, but there
are some economic, social, and psychological factors that may have combined to create that surge. Some people feel that the baby boom was related to the end of the World War II in 1945. At that time, there was an overall
optimistic mood in the country and a period of affluence in the economy.
Many women who had previously been employed to help supply the material goods necessary for the military were no longer needed. This opened the
opportunity for many of those women to leave the workplace and become
stay-at-home moms. Many young couples who were reunited began to feel
confident about the future and began having children. There was once again
easy access to consumables and higher wages for the returning GIs.

This sudden prosperity was associated with the rise of living in the sub-
urbs. Modest, inexpensive homes were being built by developers around the
urban areas, and low-cost, government-subsidized loans were readily available. The affordability of those homes and the size of the houses made it
conducive to having more children. Having a backyard and a place for these
children to play was a major factor.

Baby Boomers have been associated with the significant social changes
that they created. During the 1960s when we were teenagers, there was
great social unrest. During World War II, Americans rallied around the war
effort, but during the 1960s, there was extreme social protest on college
campuses against the American involvement in the Vietnam War, extending
even into the 1970s.

Baby Boomers tend to value relationships. As we grew up, the importance
of spending time with family and friends developed. The rapid economic

growth and increasing labor laws led to more free time. Baby Boomers are goal oriented. We have been reared with the idea of pursuing the American dream, and we push ourselves to reach our goals. Many of us are self-assured and believe that hard work makes a difference. We are resourceful and have participated in the greatest technological advances in history.

Many of us took place in the antiwar movement against American participation in Vietnam and protested with our brethren for Civil Rights for all. We were around during the beginning of the Space Race, when the Russians launched Sputnik in 1957, prompting a push for young people to enter science-related fields so the Americans would never fall behind the Russians. We watched the creation of the Berlin Wall in 1961 and the destruction of that wall in 1989. We mourned the loss of "our hero," President John F. Kennedy, who motivated many of us with his classic words, "Ask not what your country can do for you. Ask what you can do for your country."

We experienced the beginning of the Rock and Roll era and the "British Invasion" by the Beatles and the Rolling Stones. We experienced Woodstock and peace rallies all over the country.

Now, however, many of us are in our 70s and beyond. We are retired or nearly so. We are living or talk about living in condominiums in Arizona or Florida and the price of prescription drugs. Many of us spend our retirement days going to doctors on Monday, Wednesday, and Friday and prepare for those visits on Tuesday and Thursday. Another characteristic of our generation is that many of us have been much more health-conscious than our own parents. We do not smoke cigarettes as did our parents and are concerned about driving cars that are safe, and even wear helmets when we ride our bikes. Medical advances have allowed us to live longer and stay healthier than did our parents. Our parents looked at retirement as a time to relax and do nothing. We want to get out and do the things we have always dreamed of doing. We will not ever consider moving to a retirement home or even a retirement village. We do not like to think of terms like "aging" and "elderly." We want to live as long as possible but keep productive along the way. We join health clubs and keep active socially, things that our parents would have never considered.

Many of us have never taken courses in how to live a long life. Many of us do not have role models in our family who consciously took care of themselves. Many of us want to do whatever it takes to grow old gradually and gracefully, continuing to do the things we enjoy doing, not cutting back on traveling, spending money, and contributing to our community.

So, we decided to author this book for other members of the Baby Boomer generation, providing suggestions of changes to make or lifestyles to pursue to live the life we want. Feel free to read each chapter or read the ones you want. Pass on the information to others in your family or group of friends. There are no right or wrong ways to live your lives. It is purely your choice. Take all the information, assimilate it, and use it for your own needs.

This information comes from a retired physician and clinical professor and from one of the world's authorities in progressive (also called "complementary," "alternative," or "integrative") medicine or health. Collaboration in this way will provide you with information that you might not ever receive anywhere else.

As you read this book, remember that neither of us (nor any of our readers) have reached the age of 120 or even 100, yet we all want to live as long as possible, in as healthy a condition as possible, and with all our mental capabilities intact. In our professional roles, we have each have had the opportunity to interact with many centenarians (over 100 years old) who provided us with the insight on their secrets to living a long life. Our suggestions in this book are based on scientific studies that have been published, as well as our personal experiences. It would be almost impossible to develop and conduct a study of people following all our suggestions for 40 to 50 years to see how close they get to 120 years old. What we will provide you is a guide to follow, if you choose, including many suggestions, and even examples of "How to do it." These are only our suggestions for you to consider. There will be many options to choose from. Life constantly presents us with choices to make, sometimes without knowledge of what to do. Choose wisely from our suggestions; follow the ones you want to use; and ignore the others if you wish. Throughout the book, there will be text and even dialogue between us. With over 90 years of combined clinical experience working with patients, we have found that answering questions is a highly effective way of providing information to everyone, not just the person asking the question. So, we have done just that in each chapter in the book. There may be differences of opinions between us which will be obvious, but we both have the same goal—healthy and productive lives.

Each of us loves to teach and we hope that all our readers will feel like our book was written specifically for them. Enjoy reading it. We wish that all our readers will live to 120 years. Moses in the Bible lived to 120. You might do so, too.

Prologue

Aging, as we know it today, is an inevitable and unavoidable process. The aging process often brings out certain diseases that have devastating effects on our society and overloads the entire health care system and economy. These diseases include arthritis, cardiovascular disease, cancer, dementia, osteoporosis, diabetes, hypertension, tissue degeneration, neuropathy, stroke, obesity, and depression. Aging can also affect vision, hearing, muscle strength, bone mass, immunity, nerve function, and metabolic disorders. Aging is a threat to life itself and poses enormous challenges to the entire system, thereby necessitating an urgent need to address these health concerns.

Our culture and society have etched aging into our minds in a monumental way. Antibiotic discovery was the first major step. In our grandparents' generation, infectious diseases created a statistical imbalance at such an elevated level that death was early and anticipated. Antibiotics have changed that. In addition, marked improvement in infant and child mortality rates, medical advancements, fewer wars, and improved living conditions have all contributed to people living longer, yet that plateau is quite disturbing. This is easily noted in the tables below. However, please pay close attention to the plateau that has occurred for the first time in the past decade.

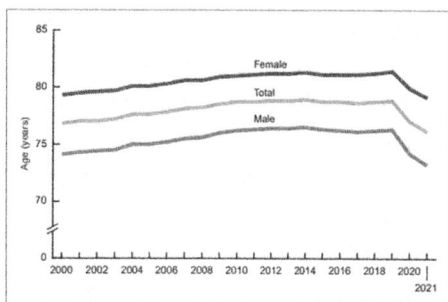

NOTES: Estimates are based on provisional data for 2021. Provisional data are subject to change as additional data are received. Estimates for 2000–2020 are based on final data.
SOURCE: National Center for Health Statistics, National Vital Statistics System, Mortality

Decade and Life Expectancy in Years		
1870 39.4	1950 67.2	2020 78.8
1880 19.4	1960 69.7	2021 77.6
1890 44.1	1970 70.3	
1900 48.2	1980 73.2	
1910 51.4	1990 74.9	
1920 53.2	2000 76.5	
1930 58.7	2010 78.2	
1940 62.0	2015 78.9	

https://www.statista.com/statistics/1040079/
life-expectancy-united-states-all-time/

Modern medicine and science have created antibiotics and vaccines, found ways to improve maternal and infant mortality, discovered and implemented modern diagnostic and treatment tools, improved living conditions, and yet that plateau is quite disturbing.

Rapidly, over the past two decades, we have found new ways to "kill ourselves." Unhealthy lifestyles slipped many of us into an abyss, laced with insanity. The leading causes of death among adults ages 65 and older are cardiovascular conditions, cancer, pneumonia, stroke, and Alzheimer's disease. For more than a decade, heart disease and cancer have been the leading causes of death in the United States. In fact, the Centers for Disease Control (CDC) has told us that the people at risk for heart disease are those who smoke, who are overweight, who have a family history of heart disease, and who have uncontrolled blood sugar levels resulting from diabetes. All those conditions are diseases of the modern lifestyle, and all were not present 50 years ago, or at least not to the degree they are being seen now. In fact, the same CDC tells us that children born today will die a minimum of 5 years sooner than their parents. As noted in the graph above, from mid-2020 to mid-2021, life expectancy fell. Despite strong antibiotic medications, more technology to help doctors diagnose problems and save lives, better insight to neonatology (medical issues around the time of birth), and pharmaceuticals for so many medical conditions, people are not continuing to live longer than they did in previous years. There is a mathematical rule regarding longevity in animals. The expected age should be seven times the length of maturity. Oversimplifying that suggests that if it takes one year for a bird to mature, the life expectancy for that bird should be seven years. If humans typically mature between ages 21 and 25, the analogy would be that they should have an expected life span of 145 to 175. Why does that not occur?

Stress, environmental toxins, inadequate nutrition, lack of sufficient exercise in our sedentary lifestyles, not enough rest, along with a plethora of other missteps, are robbing us of our vital time on Earth. Brian's personal center, Hippocrates Wellness, in West Palm Beach, FL, was established in 1956 and has been treating and monitoring thousands of patients since then. Their model has observed that changing the way people run their lives may be difficult but can lead to significant improvement in the way those people feel and impact positively on many medical conditions they may have.

But does it have to be that way? Is aging an inevitable process or do we have a chance to intervene before irreversible changes occur? Perhaps, aging is really a disease, one that can be prevented. In this book, you will read about the science behind the specific suggestions we offer. As we do so, we present practical ways to incorporate those suggestions into your lives. We have also invited experts in certain topics to contribute their knowledge to add to the impact of this book.

There is a famous prospective, observational study called "The New England Centenarian Study." The researchers in this ongoing study have tried to look at, to quantitate the subjects, and to understand why they have been able to reach the milestone of living past 100 years old. They have labeled 15% of their subjects as "escapers," 43% as "delayers," and 42% are "survivors" of demonstrable diseases. They provide some interesting demographic statistics (www.bumc.bu.edu/centenarian/statistics/) for us to consider. Out of a U.S. population in 2021, there were 89,739 centenarians (age 100+) or a prevalence of 0.27%. The prevalence of centenarians has been increasing and, in the past 20 years, the rate has nearly doubled.

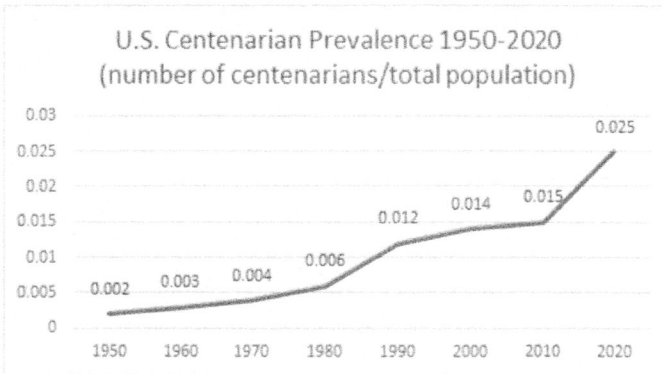

Perls T. US Centenarian Prevalence 1950-2020.

Derived from United Nations, Dept Economic and Social Affairs, Population Division (2022).

Once centenarians reach age 100, the numbers and prevalence of them drop off dramatically with increasing age. Centenarians, age 100 to 104, are found at a rate of 1 per 2,200 in our population, semi-supercentenarians are found at a rate of 1 per 34,000, and supercentenarians (over 110 years old), are found in 1 per 871,600. Interestingly, 85% of centenarians are women, and 90% of supercentenarians are women. The same group of scientists asked what do these people eventually die of? The top five causes of death were:

- Heart disease
- Alzheimer's disease
- Stroke

- Cancer
- Influenza and pneumonia

The scientists learned from their patients and their siblings that exceptional longevity runs very strongly in families.

Their comments include that health behavior choices of persons explain most of their ability or inability to reach old age. This suggests that aging can be affected by what we do to ourselves. That means to us, if you want to live longer, you need to make changes in your lives now.

Many of you know that you should make changes in your lives. This book will provide you with valuable suggestions to begin and maintain solutions to those issues.

CHAPTER 1

Healthy Eating

There are so many people on the Earth, who live in so many countries, and who are a part of so many different cultures. They all have different customs regarding food and eating. For people in poor countries, there are often insufficient amounts of food sources, so eating depends upon the availability of food and not the quality or quantity of food. For those in wealthy countries, eating is all about "choice." We will explain our observations through the windows of natural history, biology, and nutritional science. To start with, humans share the Earth with 8 million other species. In their natural settings, 100% of those animals consume raw or uncooked food. Intensive residential programs around the country have placed both healthy people and people with illnesses on a diet consisting of unprocessed and organic plant–based food and have seen specific clinical and biochemical improvements. For example, there is often seen a marked and quick return of blood sugar levels to normal in patients with poorly controlled type 2 diabetes, allowing many patients to reduce or even go off medications in a short period of time. People with known cardiovascular disease have begun to reverse their symptoms over time. Patients with painful arthritis, no longer responding to anti-arthritis medications, will frequently find improvement in symptoms within weeks of a proper diet combined with exercise and physical therapy. Science traditionally ignored these types of observations as only anecdotal, but now so many studies have confirmed the same observation, that proper attention is now being made.

The theory behind the plant-based diet goes back to the premise that every drop of energy that powers all living organisms pours down from the sun. Photons can be thought of as a gift from the sun. Evolution developed green, leafy plants that began to appear 4 million years ago. Photosynthesis became the mechanism that developed for plants to capture the photonic energy of the sun and to convert carbon dioxide and water into food, while producing oxygen as a byproduct. These living plants contain every essential nutrient that animals (including humans) require to live long without disease and environmental stresses. Over the thousands of years of human life, we have crafted our food out of ethnic preferences, flavor, and emotional satisfaction, even though food was originally meant as a fuel for our biological needs and nothing else. This is certainly the case in all animal species. Even the science of cooking is not based on biological evidence, but more on the taste of food. It is well known that the proteins in the enzymes we eat become inactivated or denatured somewhere between 100° and 120°. At that temperature range, vitamins are inactivated; proteins are disturbed; minerals are diminished; and other factors for longevity, such as hormones, oxygen, phytochemicals, and enzymes are altered. For these reasons, we emphasize the need to eat organic, unprocessed, and uncooked plant-based foods as a major part of our diets.

In certain isolated communities are tribes with collections of people who are centenarians (people over 100 years old) and super centenarians (over 110 years old) who ingest plant-based diets in their unaltered form and even consume way fewer calories than most Americans do. In addition, scientists have consistently seen an increase in the healing potential generated from empowered immunity via enzyme-rich fare. Humans are made of cells and the strength and quality they possess determines one's biological clock.

Some longevity studies focus only on genetics. The New England Centenarian Research study, sponsored by the National Institute of Aging, started in 2006, is one of the most comprehensive endeavors ever pursued that looked at genetic markers. They found 281 genetic markers that were 61% accurate in predicting who is 100 years old, 73% accurate in predicting who is 102 years old or older, and 85% accurate in predicting who is 105 years old or older. In other words, the prediction becomes more accurate with older ages and older ages beyond 100, which goes along with their hypothesis that the genetic component of exceptional longevity gets greater and greater with older and older age.

Other investigators found that food, exercise, and relationships were noted as the foundations for healthy, active aging. Holt-Lunstat *et al.* (2015) looked at people 65 years old. This study revealed that those individuals with three or four close friends added eight more years to life. CNN.com in May 2019 reviewed 148 studies that found that people who are isolated face a 50% greater risk of premature death. Social isolation carries a risk of mortality like that of smoking. Nutritional food is a cornerstone in longevity, yet it is only one of several factors that contribute. Those will be discussed in latter chapters of this book.

With all this in mind, why do we eat what we eat? Why should we make changes? If we decide to make changes, where should we start? Most importantly, what should we eat?

What determines what we eat?

Growing up, few, if any, of us received formal education or training in what to eat and why food choices are essential. We are taught how to ride a bicycle, but not what comprises healthy eating. We do not have courses on nutrition in elementary, middle, or high schools. We are bombarded by commercials for unhealthy foods, rarely by commercials to eat nutritious foods. If we are encouraged to eat a vegetarian diet, does that include potato chips and ice cream? Nutrition is rarely a college-level course, except for those individuals who choose to become nutritionists or dieticians. Even medical schools do not offer such courses.

Most of our eating habits are shaped and influenced by several factors, including the following:

- What we are fed in our families as we grow up, which is usually the same as what our parents were fed when they grew up.
- What we are fed in school lunchrooms or cafeterias or what our parents packed in our lunch boxes.
- What is available to eat at restaurants.
- What tastes good to us.
- What our friends tell us tastes good.
- What television and billboard ads promote.
- What is most convenient to eat, due to our frequent lack of time to shop and prepare food.
- What is available at local grocery stores or markets.
- What we can afford.

Even though we eat too much, too fast, and often the "wrong foods," we still survive, but not well as we could or want. It is now too easy to find takeout foods in supermarkets or even convenience stores; to buy meals at drive-through restaurants, often eating the food in the car as we drive; or to pick up lunch or dinner at fast-food restaurants because it is more convenient and less expensive than shopping at a store and then preparing food. We can order and pick up takeout food or have home-delivered food from nearly every restaurant in town, brought to us by delivery services that did not exist ten years ago. Our sedentary lifestyle has us gazing at a screen for entertainment, which has crippled our lives. With all these options, we do not have to ever leave home, and we can even eat dinner while watching TV and not even sitting at a table with our family and friends. We never change until something happens.

Voluntarily changing our diet always happens for a reason. Some of these reasons include:

- We do not like how we look in the mirror.
- We have gained weight and our clothes do not fit.
- We have an event coming up like a wedding, a reunion, a family photo-shoot, or a trip to see long-lost friends.
- We want to make ourselves look better to find a partner or a new partner.
- We are looking for a new job and know that body imagery in our society favors a certain look.
- We have recurrent stomach and intestinal symptoms always associated with eating too much of the wrong things.
- We have been diagnosed with medical conditions such as type 2 diabetes, hypertension, arthritis, heart disease, or elevated cholesterol and are advised to lose weight by our health care providers.

Clearly, the major reason that people want to change their diets is to lose weight, not necessarily to become or remain healthy. Weight loss is often viewed as a journey with a well-defined goal, such as "I need to lose 15 pounds to fit into that new suit I bought last year," or "summer is coming up and I want to look good in a bathing suit." For people of our generation, the need to lose weight is frequently driven by a medical condition that will only be reversed or improved by changing our eating habits, not by taking medications. Yet to most people, regardless of their ages, "going on a diet" implies adherence to a program for a limited period of time until that goal is reached (or close to that goal), and then returning to the same eating habits as before. It is no wonder that there is such a high incidence of recidivism (going back to the way it was) in people who suffer from obesity or weight-related illnesses. We suggest that you find a program that will teach you to eat healthy, not just to lose weight. We want you to find a program that you can remain on for the rest of your life. Losing weight will come naturally, as opposed to the goal of only losing weight regardless of what you eat or do not eat to do so.

A "fad diet" is one that becomes popular for a short time without any legitimate science to support it. These fad diets often make unreasonable claims for rapid weight loss or health improvement. In reality, there is no single definition of what comprises a "fad diet" (Wikipedia). In reality, every new fad diet is more or less just a recycled and repackaged version of an old one.

Here are some of the fad diets that have been around over the years:

Ketogenic (keto) Diet	Zone Diet	Cambridge Diet
Paleo (Paleolithic) Diet	Mayo Clinic Diet	Beverly Hills Diet
Blood-type Diet	Pritikin Diet	Rotation Diet
The Atkins Diet	Pasta Diet	Junk Food Diet
South Beach Diet	Fit for Life	Lion Diet

Each program makes claims of how effective it is and how easy it is to lose weight. Some of the diets are extremely low in fat; others are very low in carbohydrates (starches). None has proved to be sustainable over extended periods of time. Each is often associated with a book written by the creator of the diet. Sometimes, specific foods are sold to support the recommendations of the author of that diet.

Most diets tend to focus, either positively or negatively, on a select few nutrients. This is not a sound approach, as our bodies need a variety of foods. Many of today's fad diets follow a low-carbohydrate, high-protein route, without vetting the source of the protein. A review of the existing evidence (Ge *et al.,* 2020) found that limiting certain macronutrients is not more effective for weight loss in the long-term than just eating fewer calories. Low-fat or low-carbohydrate or high-protein diets—all lead to about the same amount of weight loss over a 12-month period. Participants will usually drop out of every fad diet because it is hard to follow the recommended restrictions. A meta-analysis (Powis, 2018) looked at 121 weight-loss studies and found that most people on any weight-loss diet typically did lose a significant amount of weight after 6 months but regained most of that weight in the following 6 months. Reiser (2015) found that the body resists weight loss by burning fewer calories, increasing the production of a hormone called "ghrelin" which increases appetite and decreases the production of a different hormone called "leptin," which causes the sensation of being full. The worst situation is that most published studies follow patients for only one year or less. This makes it even more difficult to know the long-term success of any diet. The conclusion of these types of studies is that any diet that a person can stay with in the long-term becomes a successful diet for that person. Powis (2019) concludes that "A healthy diet is a varied diet rich in fruits, vegetables, whole-grain products and high-quality proteins and poor in sugar, refined grains, and highly processed food." This type of diet is the easiest to follow long-term.

Because of research like this, more balanced approaches to losing weight have been created, although still associated with a commercial component.

These include Weight Watchers (which requires one to count points) or diets where you buy meals from the company (NutriSystems, Jenny Craig). Years ago, the fad was the "Protein Sparing Modified Fat" program called "Optifast" on which the famous Oprah Winfrey lost substantial weight in a brief period of time. That program abruptly terminated after some unexpected deaths.

Is there any science behind which diet is most conducive to longevity? An extremely popular diet is that of the Mediterranean diet. According to Wikipedia, the Mediterranean diet is a diet inspired by the eating habits of people who live near the Mediterranean Sea. When initially formulated in the 1960s, it drew on the cuisines of Greece, Italy, France, and Spain. In decades since, it has also incorporated other Mediterranean cuisines, such as those in Turkey, the Balkans, the Middle East, North Africa, and Portugal (Eleftherlou, 2021). The principal aspects of this diet include high consumption of olive oil, legumes, unrefined cereals, fruits and vegetables, moderate to high consumption of fish, moderate consumption of dairy products (mostly cheese and yogurt), moderate wine consumption, and low consumption of non-fish meat products. Olive oil has been studied as a potential health factor for reducing all-cause mortality and the risk of chronic diseases.

Research suggests that increasing adherence to the Mediterranean diet pattern is associated with a reduction in total and cause-specific mortality and with extending health and life span. The Mediterranean diet shares various characteristics with the similarly beneficial Okinawa diet (Wilcox, 2014). Potential anti-aging mechanisms of various nutrients are not yet understood. Shares of macronutrients and level of caloric intake may also be of significance, including periods when no dietary restriction occurs, such as not having a fat-intake that is too low and not having a prolonged caloric surplus or caloric deficit that is too large. Studies suggest dietary changes are a major cause of national relative rises in lifespan.

Adjusting the Mediterranean diet may even contribute to increased longevity. Some of those modifications include an approach to develop optimal diets for health and life span (or "longevity diets") and include:

- Modifying or further particularizing the Mediterranean diet as the baseline via nutrition science. For instance, via:
  - Additional increase in plant-based (protein-rich) food along with a corresponding restriction of meat intake (Fong et al., 2019). Meat reduction is or can be typically healthy.
  - Regular moderate consumption of green tea or (filtered) coffee while ensuring adequate calcium intake.

- Adding various foods thought to be healthy (*e.g.*, due to results about various mechanistic effects) to the regular dietary consumption patterns.
  - Increasing the intake of high-spermidine foods—studies suggest spermidine could extend life span, with high amounts of it present in fungi and green peas than in common supplements.
  - Increasing resistant starch intake—legumes, especially green peas, contain large amounts of resistant starch, especially if precooked, as cooling the cooked peas in a refrigerator substantially increases the resistant starch content due to starch retrogradation.
- Keeping alcohol consumption of any type at a minimum—conventional Mediterranean diets include alcohol consumption (*i.e.*, wine), which is under research due to data suggesting negative long-term brain impacts.
- Fully replacing refined grains—some guidelines on Mediterranean diets do not clarify or include the principle of whole-grain consumption instead of refined grains. Whole grains are a significant source of spermidine and are associated with longevity. They are the main characteristic pillar of Mediterranean diets.
- Aiming for a sufficient level of food variety and diversity—which some guidelines of Mediterranean diets do not clarify or include. One review suggests that food variety and diversity could be a factor of diet quality (Ramadas *et al.*, 2021), and another review indicates that sufficient food variety may at least in some specific cases "increase intake of important nutrients and positively affect the gut microbiome structure and function" (D'Auria *et al.*, 2020). The required level of food variety may or may not be low and vary per person and diet.
- Completely eliminating processed foods from the diet—some guidelines of Mediterranean diets may not clarify this principle. Diets associated with longevity are characterized by minimally processed foods (Campisi *et al.*, 2019).
- Adjusting the diet for personal characteristics such as age as effects of macronutrient intake can vary per age.

Our current recommendations as to the healthiest type of eating, based on the above observations, is the plant-based diet, eating foods only from plants, and eliminating all animal products, including meat, chicken, fish, eggs, dairy products, and cheese, and eating organic, unprocessed foods.

Based on our own observations and our information obtained from speaking with many others in the field, we feel that plant-based diets, also called "Vegan diets," can accomplish everything that people are looking for. When followed properly they can improve diabetes and possibly reduce heart disease, eliminate pain from arthritis, improve exercise ability, and, by the way, promote weight loss.

Why does everyone not follow a plant-based diet? These diets have been criticized for being unbalanced and too extreme because they contain no animal products. WebMD reports that non-vegans are quick to criticize those who follow plant-based eating for not having protein with each meal, for "eating grass" all the time, for eating too many carbohydrates, for not having enough omega-3 fatty acids, for having an obsession for healthy food and restriction of everything else, for not enjoying the taste of food, and for not participating in the eating of gourmet foods and alcoholic beverages.

A recent study of 63 overweight adults compared the outcomes of five different diets. Those in the plant-based group lost more than twice as much weight than those of any other groups. Other studies have shown plant-based diets may reduce several risk factors for heart disease and combined with exercise, meditation, and spirituality, may actually reverse heart disease.

We have chosen to present a great deal of information in the form of questions and answers. This format is a highly effective way to understand and process information. Many people have questions that they would not ask, but in this format, it becomes quite easy to learn. We have tried to anticipate many questions that might be considered by you.

Please keep in mind that we are only revealing many of the potential concerns that might occur when consuming certain foods and drinks. By following all our suggestions, you should be able to optimize your health. There are no data to support that following all our suggestions will guarantee increasing your life span, but they should maximize your chances of remaining in good health. As you will see throughout our writing, you should consider the advice we provide and make the best choices you can. Healthy living is all about making good choices, and good choices should maximize your chances of living a long and productive life.

Questions and Answers

1. How do you define a plant-based diet?

Plant-based diets include vegetables, fruits, nuts, seeds, grains, and beans. They specifically exclude any animal derived "fare." Ideally, the food is organic, leaving behind the potential disease-causing chemicals that pervade commercial agriculture. When possible, consuming the least processed and uncooked varieties of these botanical choices preserves their nutrients and medicinal properties.

2. *What is organic food? What adverse effects can be caused by food additives, herbicides/pesticides, and preservatives?*

"Organic food" and organic everything else is quite the fad now. There are organic restaurants, organic eggs, organic chickens, organic dry cleaners, organic clothes, and many other stores front advertising their "organic" products.

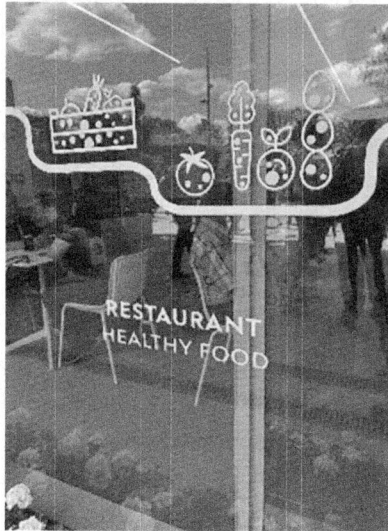

Organic food is grown in rich, nutritious soil, without the assistance of chemical fertilizers, pesticides, or fungicides. In many regions of the world, governments have stringent rules to what is allowed to be labeled as "organic/biodynamic/ecological." "Biodynamic" has even stricter criteria than "organic." Biodynamic is from the Rudolf Steiner (www.waldorfeducation.org) school of thought and is ecologically balanced. Consumption of "food" which contains certain manmade chemicals (including most herbicides, pesticides, fungicides, heavy metals, pharmaceutical drugs, and even plastic) can disturb the cellular function of our bodies, potentially activating neurological or hormonal problems. Cancer may be directly tied to consumption of such "food." In the United States, there is a 5-digit numbering system for categorizing food.

Stickers are on each vegetable or fruit sold with a number. All organic food starts with the number "9" followed by four additional digits. Most states adhere to extremely strict guidelines in allowing the use of the organic indication of "9."

Preservation of food has become a major industry, as food is often transported from one part of the country to another and often may remain on a grocery store shelf or even a refrigerator for days to weeks without a consumer ever being aware of it. These preservatives can play havoc on the digestive and elimination systems. Over the years, many such preservatives have been scientifically questioned or actually removed from the marketplace because of their toxic effects. These include Red Dye #2, Yellow Dye #4, and Carrageenan. Carrageenan has been implicated in causing gastrointestinal cancers in animals and may have the same effect in humans. Tartrazine Yellow #5 has been widely used in the food and pharmaceutical industry but has been reported to cause hyperactivity in some young children and occasionally skin allergy in adults.

Benzophenone, ethyl acrylate, methyl eugenol are all compounds that are petrochemical in origin and are used in food products or food packaging. Benzophenone has been banned in the United States. Breast cancer has been associated with the consumption of these products. Additional chemicals that have been banned include eugenol methyl ether (methyl eugenol), myrcene, pulegone, and pyridine.

Even though cases of medical issues have been reported, relating to consumption of foods containing the above chemicals used in their production or preservation, there is no guarantee that eating these will cause you, as an individual, to become ill in any way. By eating only organic products, however, you minimize your risk of exposure to these products. Remember, healthy eating is all about making good choices.

3. Do calories matter?

Calories are historically a unit of energy. Scientists have defined "calorie" to mean a unit of energy or health that could come from a variety of sources such as coal or gas. In a nutritional sense, all types of food (carbohydrates, fat, proteins) are important sources of calories that people need to live and function.

In our society, weight loss is always connected with reduction of calories more than what a person needs to live on to regulate baseline body function (digestion, heart beating, breathing, and elimination), plus whatever is used up in muscle work (such as doing exercise).

Unfortunately, the type of calories in healthy versus unhealthy foods determines the benefit of eating. For example, a slice of white bread may have a lower caloric count than a piece of fresh fruit. The body has an innate ability to determine which fuel is most appropriate for its function. Obviously, the fruit "wins." This view contrasts to when scientists thought of food as pure energy without the consideration of the nutrients that food provides for vitality and longevity.

4. *Are foods like ice cream, frozen yogurt, Greek yogurt, French fries, potato chips, and bagels considered plant-based?*
   Although these "food choices" are universally adored, they do not promote health and, in fact, are linked to a wide variety of diseases. Yogurt marketers wisely promote the "benefits" of the healthy bacteria that yogurt contains or the calcium-rich milk which is the base of all dairy products. However, there is consensus among researchers internationally that all previous understanding of the essential attitude of consuming these products is more "sales than it is science." In fact, these so-called healthy choices are linked to heart disease, cancer, diabetes, osteoporosis, and more.

   French fries, potato chips, and pretzels (among many other foods) taste good and do contain high concentrations of plant-based carbohydrates. However, they all contain potential carcinogens (cancer promoters). During the process of turning the potatoes into food an element called "acrylamide" is produced. According to the Food and Drug Administration (FDA) acrylamide is formed through a natural chemical reaction between sugars and asparagine, an amino acid, in plant-based foods—including potato and cereal-grain foods. Acrylamide forms during high-temperature cooking such as frying, roasting, and baking. In research studies, elevated levels of acrylamide caused cancer in laboratory animals, but the levels of acrylamide used in those studies were much greater than those found in human food. The FDA has been closely monitoring this contaminant for years and has encouraged growers, manufacturers, and food service operators to reduce acrylamide in the food supply.

5. *What is wrong with drinking regular soda, diet soda, or even flavored carbonated water?*
   Common soda begins with unclean water and progresses poorly from there. Some of those drinks are quite full of sugar as well as carbonation.

Some people feel that carbonation may impede the oxygen-carrying capacity of the blood. In addition, most soft drinks contain synthetic flavoring, dyes, stabilizers, and are distributed in either plastic bottles or in aluminum cans. If we were to invent something bad for your health, we could not do a better job. Diet-drinks add new dimensions to their noxiousness by relying on chemicals such as aspartame, which is noted for its neurological and brain derogating elements. Beverage companies shrewdly recognize a growing trend toward health and now offer such nonsensical drinks like "vitamin water." The chemically created supplements that are added to water offer little nutritional value, but the artificial sweetener that they spike it with does the same damage that this substance is known for. Tucker *et al.* (2006) suggested that it was phosphoric acid, which is the coloring agent for cola drinks, that may be associated with low bone mineral density.

6. *What substance in milk is harmful? Is it the sugar, the lactose, the fat, or casein?*

Milk and its derivatives (cheese, butter, cream, whipped cream, yogurt, ice cream, and kefir) contain different amounts of "poison." In the United States, as well as in other countries, there are laws allowing up to 750,000 bacterial cultures in one cup of milk. It is not a natural process to consume milk from another species. In fact, humans are the only species that consume milk after weaning. However, not every human consumes milk or milk products. Asians, for example, never drink milk.

Bacteria are also present in dairy products, including butter, cheese, and yogurt. Lactose is a natural sugar contained in cow's milk that may contribute to the development of certain autoimmune diseases, specifically type 1 diabetes. It may be the cow's insulin that triggers the immune reaction. In addition, a large percentage of our population is intolerant to lactose, resulting in abdominal pains and loose stool after consumption. Saturated fat, which is contained in all dairy products, has "clogging potential" that is linked to everything from acne to arthritis. Finally, there is casein. In the late 20th century, a profound discovery at Cornell University exposed this protein that is found in milk as the greatest contributor to atherosclerotic heart disease and maybe cancer. Michaelsson *et al. (2014)* from Uppsala University in Sweden highlights that one glass of milk a day can reduce life span by up to 15% along with showing an increased risk of hip fracture in separate cohorts of women and men. The authors hypothesized that the d-galactose in milk that might cause the problem as d-galactose is thought to induce changes that resemble natural aging. DeBoer *et al.* (2015) showed that preschoolers who are given low-fat (1%) milk, as recommended by the American Academy of Pediatrics, are more likely to be overweight or obese than children given 2% or whole milk and, over time, gain weight at a similar rate as children drinking 2% or whole milk. This shows that it is not just the fat and sugar that may contribute to weight gain, but there are other elements that might contribute as well.

7. *Should oil be eaten? What is the difference between vegetable oil, olive oil, safflower oil, pumpkin oil, sesame oil, and avocado oil? Can all be eaten? If so, how much?*

All oils should be consumed as organic cold-pressed (non-heated) varieties. These include walnut oil, avocado oil, macadamia oil, chia oil, and olive oil among others. If one has a history of atherosclerotic heart disease, that person should minimize the consumption of additional oil as oil is thought to be atherogenic. One can derive the necessary omega oils from consumption of seeds, nuts, and sprouts. In all cases, oil should be consumed sparingly. The Italians invented a device called the "Misto Can" in which you place oil in a can, then pump the spray so that a very light mist can then permeate your salad if you use oil as a salad dressing. Try not to use oil in cooking, as it is known to promote heart concerns as well as possibly contribute to cancer. Other ways to cook food include baking, steaming, or air frying. Omega-3, Omega-6, and Omega-9 oils are what most health professionals focus on. DHEA is essential to nervous system function. You may want to assure the acquisition of this by taking plant-based supplements of DHEA.

8. *If you do not suffer from heart disease, high blood pressure, or kidney problems, why is consuming salt so bad?*

Sodium is an essential mineral that human bodies require to maintain fluid balance. It is not only an electrolyte, but it also helps to cleanse the lymphatic glands, the reginal epicenter of immune cell development and the major filter system that graces every part of your anatomy. Organic sodium is derived from celery and its juices and/or sea vegetables that have been rinsed, for example, which are some of the best sources of naturally occurring sodium. Table salt, which is a highly processed form of sodium, only offers the dehydration and coagulation effect of reducing blood flow in your vascular system. This may be why blood pressure goes higher when consuming salt. Other varieties like Celtic salt, Himalayan salt, black salt, sea salt, and pink salt, have added nutrients in their composition, yet are still sodium chloride, which is the same as table salt. Some scientists do feel that so long as an individual does not knowingly have dehydration, hypertension, heart disease, or kidney disease, consumption of salt is not a problem.

9. Are eggs part of a plant-based diet?

Eggs are now being marketed as "Real Food," after noting an ever-increasing decline in egg consumption. The industry reengaged the public in a way that seemingly worked. Consuming eggs, which are unborn chickens, not only has the same disadvantages for your well-being as consuming their adult counterparts, but they are even more hazardous when it comes to cholesterol and possibly to contamination with *Salmonella* and *E. coli*. Chousalkar *et al.* (2017) found a significant incidence of *Salmonella enteritidis* in egg and egg products associated with food-born outbreaks in the United States and the United Kingdom. One egg contains 230 grams of cholesterol. Healthy individuals are not required to eat any cholesterol, since our own bodies produce this essential lipid. Egg consumption seems to contribute to many major diseases and, therefore, might shorten life span. This might be caused by the consumption of an amino acid, choline, which seems to be present in egg yolks. Choline has been reported (Martinez del Campo, 2015) to interact with gut bacteria and for trimethylamine N-oxide (MRAO) which increases blood cells' tendency to clot. This amino acid chain can reduce the flow of blood to the brain and the heart.

Egg whites are often touted as a healthier choice, because the yolk of the egg contains the cholesterol. However, consuming egg whites, no differently than consuming the entire egg, will still contain choline, although not as much. In addition, egg whites can still contain the same *Salmonella* and E. coli bacteria that are often found in whole eggs.

10. Can you snack on popcorn, either air-popped or microwaved?

Although popcorn is a highly heated food which may contain acrylamides, this is a relatively healthy occasional snack compared to most others. An air-popped type of popcorn is preferred as the corn is not popped in heated oil. There are many herbal seasonings and even plant-based butter substitutes, which can be used to replace the noxious chemicals contained in some flavorings. Microwaved popcorn is very popular, because it is so convenient, but it should never be eaten according to some experts who feel that microwaving may destroy certain nutrients in food.

11. Should all food we eat be uncooked ("raw")? What does cooking do to vegetables?

When people are attempting to reverse a major health challenge like cancer, it is a 100% organic, plant-based, raw diet is suggested to be followed for a period of time. When healthy and strong, up to 25% of one's diet by weight, can be cooked, using less destructive cooking methods like lightly steaming, air frying, and baking. This percentage has risen because of an observational study (unpublished) conducted in 1983 at Tufts University. They found that in healthy people, the immune system was not compromised until the person started consuming more than 25% of their food as cooked.

Cooking food destroys vitamins, alters the amino acid/protein chains, and reduces the amount of minerals in the food. It also destroys hormones, oxygen in the cells of plants, and phytochemicals in the same plants, as well as deactivating enzymes. These are some of the most important medicinal properties of plant-based foods. Remember, humans are the only species in the world that consumes cooked food.

In addition, three landmark studies have been published. The first, from the Pasteur Institute in Paris, demonstrated that heating food engages the white blood cells to attack the food, thereby reducing the immunological cells that are available to protect you from certain disorders. This process is called "leukocytosis." The second study, also from the Pasteur Institute, was released in the 1950s, and linked cooking to cardiovascular disease and cancer. The last Pasteur study showed that acrylamides are carcinogens derived from highly heated carbohydrates such as potatoes, breads, cereals, and other vegetable and grain products. These acrylamides may be the toxin associated with heating or cooking food.

The suggestion, therefore, is to try to eat as much raw (uncooked) food as possible, but be realistic that 25% or maybe even 50% cooked is certainly better for you than all cooked.

12. *Where should one buy vegetables? What if there are no sources of organic vegetables that are either available or affordable? Is it worse to eat fresh "nonorganic" vegetables or buy frozen vegetables?*

The concept of organic, locally grown food is spreading globally. In many areas of the country are farmers' markets at which locally grown fresh fruits and vegetables are available for at least part of the year. Your grocery stores might offer some organic vegetables, although you never know when the produce was picked or harvested. We understand that many people do not have easy access to organic foods. If you have limited access to organic produce, you might focus on the items that contain the most pesticides and herbicides and avoid those. A list has been prepared by the Environmental Working Group (EWG) (see Question 30), which publishes each year a list of the "Dirty Dozen" and "Clean Fifteen" fruits and vegetables tracked according to pesticide content.

Increasing numbers of companies now ship organic food directly to your home. As of 2023, these include Thrive Market, Misfits Market, Imperfect Foods, Butcherbox, Public Goods, and even Amazon Prime. Be aware that even though they sell "organic" food, it does not mean that everything for sale on these sites is healthy. Also, remember that for you, ambitious people who have time on your hands, you can easily grow your own sprouts, the most nutritious food available on earth, using jars and trays in your house or apartment. These germinated nut seeds, grains, and beans contain complete proteins, and all the vitamins and minerals needed for health. Sprout and microgreen growers are spread throughout the world. If you are not ambitious enough to grow your own food or feel you do not have the skills to do so, you might be able to find a company that will help you. Many people choose to have these fruits and vegetables delivered to them or have them available for curbside pickup.

What about buying frozen vegetables if there are no other choices? Fresh food, especially if you can buy them directly from a farmer, at a local market, or from a food co-op where a group of health-conscious individuals who band together to obtain foods from a farmer and distribute them to other co-op members, is always the best. We realize that people who live in urban areas may not have those opportunities. Some supermarkets or grocery stores have a limited number of choices, especially in parts of town where eating healthy is not popular and food often sits on the produce shelves for a while without being sold. We do want our readers to shift their food choices to include more vegetables and fruits, so we must consider frozen options when there are no other choices. In general, frozen foods retain their vitamins and minerals, and there is no change in the carbohydrate, protein, or fat content. Certain brands are even labeled as "frozen organic food." Be careful, however, because some of the same companies also sell "organic sausage," "organic chicken," and "organic bone broth." Often, their claims of being "organic" are not substantiated.

Just keep in mind that your food choices should have a priority: organic, directly obtained from a grower, organic from an organic market, organic from a food co-op, organic from the organic section of a food store, fresh but not organic, frozen. Keep these facts in mind as you shop for your food.

13. *Sprouts are an important part of the plant-based program. Where can one find the myriad of sprouts that are available? Stores like Whole Foods sometimes sell sprouts, but it is never known how long they have been in the vegetable section of the store. What should you do if you cannot sprout seeds yourself or grow them in a tray in soil? What do you do in the winter? If you can only find a few sprouts, which ones should you chose?*

Sprouts and microgreens are amazing sources of nutrients, including proteins, vitamins, and minerals. Some sprouts/microgreens can be found in supermarkets globally. The traditional mung bean sprout (Chinese bean sprout) is rich in protein and zinc, a mineral that helps to maintain natural hair color and fight common colds by promoting the body's natural immune system. Alfalfa and clover sprouts are commonly available and are said to help strengthen blood cells; cleanse the lungs, liver, kidneys, and bladder; and, most importantly, also afford an adaptive immune system support. Other sprouts such as sunflower sprouts, pea sprouts, onion sprouts, fenugreek sprouts, and broccoli sprouts are also amazing sources of protein and other nutrients but are rarely found in grocery stores. They must be purchased at a farmer's market or at a sprout grower. Many sprout growers do ship. A Google Search of "sprout growers near me" might yield new places for you to buy your sprouts.

If you can grow an outdoor garden in a small space at home, you can produce crops every few days that can nourish you, your family, and your friends, with the healthiest forms of food today. Ideally you grow or purchase a variety that will assure a comprehensive nutritional profile.

If you are just buying one, start with sunflower microgreens, the second alfalfa, the third, maybe, mung, the fourth may be onion, and the list continues. There is no seed that cannot be grown into a powerful healing and nourishing food for little money and even less effort.

At one time, obstetricians advised pregnant women to avoid sprouts because of possible *Salmonella* contamination. *Salmonella* is a cause of infectious diarrhea. Subsequently, there have been no other reports of that bacterium infesting sprouts. Sprouts continue to be a wonderful source of proteins, vitamins, and minerals.

14. **Why are animal products so bad for you? Is it the composition of the amino acids in the proteins of meat? Is it the animal fat that is always associated with the animal protein? Is it a contamination of substances used in raising the animals, such as antibiotics, hormones, or other chemicals used to promote rapid growth of the animal?**
Hamblin (2019) explored some of the key issues. "Global meat production has grown by five times since the 1960s. Globally, meat consumption is projected to increase by 75% over the next three decades.

"Experts have long disagreed about the exact contribution of eating meat to health, with advocates of abstinence and inundation at the tail ends of the curve. Through it all, though, Americans have always eaten more than any mainstream guideline has ever recommended.

"For most of history, in much of the world, meat eating was synonymous with prosperity. Wealthy people who could eat meat constantly grew tall and strong, and the poor subsisted on porridge and potatoes, or starved. That rapidly changed in the mid-20th century, as some wealthy countries developed the agricultural and transportation technology to make fast food cheap and ubiquitous. Chain restaurants, government subsidies, and a jingoistic idea that meat is synonymous with America have ensured that consumption has grown decade over decade."

Coinciding with the rise in the consumption of meat and other processed foods, heart disease surpassed infectious diseases as the leading cause of death in wealthy countries. Attempting to stem the tide, people started thinking about what they ate. Taking a nutrient-focused approach, most experts targeted one or two compounds as the possible cause of (or solution to) all our health concerns. Some experts recommended avoiding cholesterol and saturated fat. The American Heart

Association even endorsed a "low-fat" diet in 1961. Others supported Atkins-style dieting, essentially the opposite, beginning in the 1960s. Today "paleo," "keto," and "low carb" advocates continue to tell followers that the establishment scientists have lied to them about meat's dangers and promote eating more saturated fat and cholesterol. Whom should you believe? Are there any scientific studies to provide us with guidelines?

With something like diet, a randomized controlled trial is extremely difficult. It is impossible to have blinded subjects (people know what they're eating) or to ask people to change their entire diet for decades. As a result, most nutritional evidence is based on observational studies: looking at large groups of people over time and seeing how their diet relates to their health. In that model, it is possible to identify patterns, but it is never possible to say with absolute certainty which element of a diet is responsible for which outcome.

We, therefore, cannot show a study that compares meat eaters to vegetarians, controlling for so many variables and continued for 15 to 20 years. We can only present information and suggestions. We will never insist that longevity is only achieved with a flesh-free diet, even though we believe it ourselves.

One theory is that animal products inherently contain three erosive acids—eicosapentaenoic acid (EPA), docosapentaenoic acid (DPA), and docosahexaenoic acid (DHA)—which are not congruent with our digestive and illumination canal and, sadly, leave behind fatty debris (Rosell *et al.*, 2005). These are bioaccumulative toxins that are ingested over a lifetime. These toxins are not only found in flesh (red meat, poultry, pork, fish, and other seafood) but also in milk and all the "dairy products" that are manufactured from milk. Another theory is that human antibiotic resistance may directly come from consuming animal products and the antibiotics that were injected into them while they were growing. Estrogens and growth-promoting hormones are employed in both male and female animals to fatten them up, since meat is sold by the pound/kilo, and farmers stand to make more money with larger animals. We feel that there is no real need to consume animal products, certainly to the extent that most Americans consume them. This information is consistent with the observations made on the health of populations globally. Some scientists also feel that animal fat is atherogenic (causes hardening of the arteries), and casein in milk may also contribute to heart disease. There are even anecdotal reports that removing animal products from one's diet helps improve the aches and joint pains commonly referred to as "arthritis."

15. ***How do you feel about other types of frozen entrees such as "fake" burgers, "chick-burgers," veggie-bacon, veggie-sausage, or other frozen items?***

When one is first embracing improvement in their food choices, a bridge is necessary in the majority of cases. For this reason, organic selections of frozen food, including plant-derived burgers and "taste-alike" chicken, are good first steps. As we say above, fresh unprocessed foods would still be better. Those who are in the conquest of disease must try to obtain the maximum nutrition and medicinal potency from unprocessed, raw, vegan choices. Once a woman or a man commits to bringing about her or his own recovery, adding a small amount of cooked organic plant fare to the diet, psychologically and socially, makes things easier. Be cautious that all of you never over-consume what does not have the same benefit as a pure fresh vegan diet.

16. ***Why is tofu so bad? Are other types of soy products, like edamame, healthy to eat?***

Tofu is not meat, but it is often promoted as a meat substitute. In the process of producing this soy product, the soybeans are heated to extremely high temperatures, then formed into a square, packaged, and sold in a supermarket. Eventually this product is heated again at home before it is eaten. Remember, tofu has no taste of its own and absorbs what it is cooked in. Another potential problem with consumption of soy products is that soy products that we can buy are all GMO (genetically modified organism or food). A GMO food is any whole food whose genetic material has been altered using genetic engineering techniques. Typically, a gene from another food or living organism is implanted into the food's DNA to give it more desirable properties. Some types of genetic modification in plants have been used for thousands of years by farmers, including cross-pollinating plants and root grafting. Genetic modification is used to make crops more resistant to drought, pests, or disease, and, in some cases, to improve the taste, size, or nutrition of the plant. Genetically engineered crops also have helped to decrease the cost of food production for farmers and have reduced greenhouse gas emissions. The safety of GMO foods has always been controversial. Because the FDA does not consider GMOs different from other foods, that organization considers that GMO products are safe for human consumption. Some of the "unexpected effects" and health risks posed by GMO foods include:

- Toxicity
- Allergic reactions
- Antibiotic resistance
- Immunosuppression
- Cancer
- Loss of nutrition

A specific comment needs to be made about soymilk consumption and estrogen levels in women. There are very weak data to suggest that plant-based estrogens in soy may lower estrogen levels, but that is still controversial.

As with all our comments, the decision to eat tofu (soy) is up to you.

17. Is microwaved food so bad for you?

Microwave cooking uses frequencies that disturb the molecular structure of the food you are heating. Heating food this way is quick and easy. Because the body contains a large amount of water, exposure to direct, intense microwaves can cause tissues to heat up which could result in damage and burns. Most microwave ovens used at home are safe. If the door to the microwave is broken or damaged, radiation can leak out. If you superheat water beyond its boiling point, the water will not appear to boil, but as soon as you add something to the water in a mug, for example, instant coffee, it may suddenly boil or even explode. If the water spills over the edge of a mug, severe burns can occur. Never microwave food or infant's milk in a plastic container.

Microwaves are often said to deplete nutrients out of food but that may not be true. In fact, research from as far back as the 1980s shows that microwaved food has only slight nutritional differences from stove-cooked food. Mostly, microwaves cause extra moisture loss, which makes your food dry.

Additionally, microwaves might stop some nutrient loss. Heating and cooking food can cause nutrients to break down. The longer something is heated, the more degradation that happens. Microwaves have a shorter cooking time, though, and this stops some of the nutrient breakdown. Take Vitamin C, for example. Vitamin C in microwaved foods is preserved better than foods cooked in a regular oven.

18. *What about drinking water and water used in cooking? Is there a difference between the types of water you can consume?*
    What is the difference between these?

- Tap water
- Spring water
- Distilled water
- Purified water
- Deionized water

- Reverse osmosis water
- Carbon-filtered water
- Ultrafiltered water
- Ultraviolet oxidized water

Tap water usually comes from local rivers or underground aquifers. This water is usually processed with basic filtration techniques like flocculation, which adds chemicals to the water to get floating particles to coagulate so that they can be removed; sand filtration, which filters out large pieces of debris; or chlorination, which adds chlorine to kill bacteria and other microorganisms.

Tap water is considered drinkable by the Environmental Protection Agency (EPA), but it still can lead to numerous problems. Chlorine, for example, is not ideal for human consumption. While our bodies can usually handle chlorine, it can lead to a series of health complications and is potentially carcinogenic. This is described in a U.S. EPA publication (https://www.epa.gov/sites/default/files/2016-09/documents/chlorine.pdf).

Lead contamination also presents a risk due to lead being present in the water pipes carrying water into one's home or into a restaurant. Tap water may also contain other dissolved solids, including fertilizers in some parts of the country, and even more. Tap water may be the least expensive form of drinking or water used in cooking, but it comes with some potential issues. If you are concerned about chemicals in your food, then you might look for alternatives to ordinary tap water.

Spring water is often mistaken for being equal or interchangeable with purified water. However, spring water often contains many of the same impurities found in well or tap water. In fact, since springs feed our rivers, there is a lot of spring water in our tap water! Spring water generally has the same total dissolved solids range as tap water.

Many spring water companies advertise their water as "100% pure," but if it's not purified, what does that mean? The "pure" part refers to the source, not the water itself—in that 100% of that bottle's contents came from an underground source (rather than surface water). This clever wording leads many people to believe that spring water is just as clean as purified water.

Thanks to this crafty marketing, spring water often conjures up natural, pleasant imagery. Most spring water is not actually bottled at the source, but rather, is pumped into large tanker trucks from the source to be transported to the bottling facility. The water in those trucks must always contain chlorine or ozone to protect against contamination. In this sense, spring water is hardly different from tap water. Once the water is at the bottling facility, it goes through a carbon filtration process to remove the chlorine. This process may separate spring from tap water, but nitrates, metals, and more are likely to remain.

Distilled water is processed by boiling water (H_2O) out of its contaminants. Many of these contaminants include inorganic minerals or metals. Those impurities have a much higher boiling point than water's boiling point of 212 °F. So, the steam that results from the boiling is captured and cooled—and the water that results from the steam is what is classified as distilled water. Because many of the volatile compounds in water have a lower boiling point than water, they boil off first. As a result, it is important to employ additional purification methods beyond distillation to have truly clean, pure water.

Filtered water is what you are most likely to find in a grocery store. It is typically sourced from municipal tap water, which is then run through carbon filters to remove the chlorine (which improves the taste) and sometimes a micron filter as well. After the filtering, it is ozonated and bottled. In essence, filtered water is quite like spring water. It comes from a "natural" source, goes through minimal filtration, and is then bottled and shipped to market.

Purified water is all about the purification methods that separate purified water from the rest of the pack. Purified water goes through a process similar to what filtered water goes through, but with a few added steps like reverse osmosis, distillation, or deionization. The result is far purer than filtered, spring, or tap water.

Deionized water is purified water that has had almost all of its mineral ions removed, such as calcium, sodium, iron, copper, chloride, and sulfate. The process to produce this uses specially manufactured ion-exchange resins that exchange hydrogen (H^+) and hydroxyl (OH^-) molecules ions for dissolved minerals and then recombine to form H_2O.

Reverse Osmosis (RO) is the reverse of the naturally occurring process of osmosis. Osmosis is the movement of water molecules from low ion concentration to high ion concentration through a semiperme-able membrane. The osmotic process is used by our cells to maintain osmotic balance of the intercellular environment(s). The method of producing RO water is a simple matter of applying increased pressure to one side of the system. By applying additional pressure to one side, in this case the untreated or dirtier water side, feed-water is forced through semipermeable membranes resulting in more purified water. The RO process can typically remove 90–99% of contaminants. Al-though not perfect, RO purification is a cost-effective method because if used properly RO membranes can last for years. You can have an RO device in your house, or you can buy RO water in places like Amazon. com, Target, Walgreens, Kroger, and Whole Foods, among others, as of 2023.

Carbon-filtered water is formed by using carbon block filters made of a solid block of compressed carbon and are often used as a pre-filter in RO and other water filtration systems. These filters are extremely effec-tive in filtering out a variety of contaminants.

Ultrafiltered water is made by using a variety of membrane filtration in which hydrostatic pressure forces a liquid against a semipermeable membrane. Suspended solids and solutes of high molecular weight are retained, while water and low-molecular-weight solutes pass through the membrane.

Ultraviolet oxidized water uses ultraviolet rays to kill the harmful bac-teria from the water. Hence, the water is completely disinfected from pathogens. Ultraviolet water is good for health because it kills all the harmful microbes present in the water without affecting the taste.

So, what type of water you should you drink? The EWG warned that millions of Americans are unwittingly drinking water that includes an invisible toxic cocktail made up of contaminants linked to cancer, brain damage, and other serious health harms. The various forms of purified or filtered water can be purchased in stores or ordered online. The choice is ultimately yours. When possible, choose water that comes in glass bottles or nontoxic metal bottles rather than water in plastic bot-tles, not because of the fear of plastic in the water, but to cut down on plastic pollution to our environment.

We feel that you should choose between drinking distilled water or RO water. Since it is difficult to find RO water in supermarkets or other stores, and very easy to find distilled water, the choice of water is often that of distilled water.

One-half ounce of water per pound of body weight of pure fluid is the general rule of how much one requires each day. A 100-pound person would need to consume 50 ounces per day. Of course, you must take into consideration athletic activity, warmer climates, work environments, and exercise levels. Water not only makes up most of your body weight but is the most lubricant allowing plasma to effortlessly move throughout your body. On the vanity front, more water equals fewer wrinkles.

Whether you can safely drink carbonated water is controversial. Tucker *et al.* (2006) looked at 2,500 men and women who consumed soft drinks and carbonated water. Cola drinks contain caffeine and phosphoric acid and were associated with significantly lower bone mineral density at each hip, but not the spine in women, but no changes in men. These drinks do contain acids and sugars and can cause erosion of the enamel of teeth and tooth decay, especially if consumed in large quantities.

The process of carbonation is simply the addition of pressurized carbon dioxide gas to plain water. There is a misconception that carbon dioxide gas, dissolved in carbonated water as carbonic acid, is highly acidic and can damage teeth; however, a 2012 study failed to demonstrate any effects on tooth enamel (The Truth about Sparkling Water and Your Teeth | Mouth Healthy—Oral Health Information from the ADA).

Carbonation may cause bloating and gas, which can cause a flare-up of irritable bowel syndrome. Carbonation, per se, does not seem to have any detrimental effects, but adding flavors that contain sodium, natural and artificial acids, flavors, sweeteners, and other additives can be a problem.

One special area of water solutes that needs to be discussed is that of fluoride. The Centers for Disease Control (CDC) maintains that community water fluoridation is safe. Fluoride has been added to community water supplies since the 1940s throughout the United States to prevent tooth decay, which it has done. Now, however, in an era of fluoridated toothpastes and other consumer products that "boost dental health," the potential risks from consuming fluoridated water may outweigh the benefits for some people. In 2015, the U.S. Public Health Service lowered its recommended levels of fluoride in drinking water (Public Health Reports, 2015). Fluoride may be toxic at high levels. Excessive fluoride causes "fluorosis," which is erosion of tooth enamel that ranges from barely noticeable white spots to staining and pitting. Fluoride can also accumulate in the calcification front of newly forming bone, altering the bone's structure and maybe even weakening the skeleton. Also, some data in laboratory animals suggest that high levels of fluoride may be toxic to brain and nerve cells. Some epidemiological studies have identified possible links to learning, memory, and cognition deficits, though most of those studies were from populations with higher fluoride than in most U.S. cities.

The answers are still not in as to whether adding fluoride to water, or even to toothpaste, to prevent dental cavities outpaces the risks to bone or nervous system cells. As in other recommendations, we leave the choice up to you.

19. *Some Doctors often recommend fish, as a choice over chicken or beef/lamb/pork. What is wrong with that?*

Fish and fish oil have been promoted as "healthier foods." The surplus oil that cost handsome money to discard became a source of income for the supplement industry. Consumption of fish, such as salmon, often touted as rich in omega oils, is presumably very heart healthy. Ironically, most fish are raised in factory farms and exposed to dyes, antibiotics, and the discards of the fellow fish packed into a small tightly packed area. Some studies (Lombardi *et al.,* 2021; Aung *et al.*, 2018; McCarty, *et al.*, 2014) have linked fish and fish oil consumption to cardiovascular disease, including atrial fibrillation, and prostate cancer. When a conventional physician advises you to eat poultry, rather than red meat, they are leading you into a higher incident of a wide variety of disorders. Fatty lamb and pork are even more culpable in the creation of illness and premature death. When people consume these flesh-based choices today, the vast majority know that it is not the best yet decide to continue it despite that knowledge and supportive research. There is no doubt that it is hard to break patterns, and there is enough misinformation flying around to give you the support you search for in continuing on this path to a shorter life span.

20. *Can I eat potatoes? What is the difference between white potatoes and sweet potatoes? Are there any differences between the several types of white potatoes and the various types of sweet potatoes?*

White potatoes, with their high starch content, are not good plant-based foods. Other potatoes, from uniquely different family, such as sweet potatoes and yams, happen to be highly nutritious root vegetables that most people can consume without concern. Those people who have diabetes should avoid any sugar-rich food until they bring their blood sugar levels into control. Air-fried sweet potatoes are becoming popular, and you should make that selection whenever possible.

21. ***What is the problem with eating sugar? What about maple syrup, honey, or agave? What artificial sweeteners are acceptable?***

Sugar is one of the most addictive substances known to man. Generations of industries have spiked their food with this crystal knowing that those who consume it will be seduced into buying their products repeatedly. Although we have been trained to believe that other forms of sugar like honey, maple syrup, and agave are better, there is no validity to this claim. The medical archives now contain a plethora of supportive data that point to the erosive and disease-expanding properties of all forms of sugar (Yang *et al.*, 2014). Needless to say, sugar may also add additional undesired calories and fat to your body.

22. ***Are alcohol, beer, or wine acceptable to consume? If so, which one of these is "better"? How much alcohol is acceptable to consume?***

All alcohol has the same chemical composition. Smaller amounts of alcohol are contained in beer and higher amounts in spirits. Unscrupulous industry marketers have employed scientists to fabricate bogus studies that made claims of the benefit alcohol consumption affords. In recent years, legitimacy has begun to emerge with clear, descriptive, findings that "there is no healthy level of alcohol." As a side note, alcohol can literally be called "liquid sugar," and its main addictive quality is just that. If alcohol destroys the liver and brain cells in large amounts, does it not do the same in smaller amounts?

A relatively low incidence of heart disease reported in French people is often attributed to the consumption of red wine. Red wine contains resveratrol which may reduce cardiovascular disease and heart failure. One can take resveratrol medication instead of drinking red wine if that is your belief.

23. ***What is the difference between being a "vegetarian," being a "vegan," being a "rawtarian," and being on a "plant-based diet"?***

Vegetarians often consume plant-based foods, but many will include eggs and dairy in what they eat. "Pure" vegetarians are now called "vegans" and consume no animal products at all. Plant-based diets vary in categories of cooked, partially raw, or totally raw. Additionally, many vegans will consume processed foods that are not often healthy. An emerging group of people consider themselves vegans but call themselves "pescatarians" because they also choose to eat fish. Unfortunately, fish, especially farmed fish, is often riddled with pesticides and contains the same undesirable saturated fat that is contained in steak, butter, or even whipped cream. The last group is the "rawtarians," who consume only organic, unprocessed, uncooked plant foods with more of an emphasis on green vegetables and less on fruit. The latter way of eating is often extremely hard to sustain without maximal effort and socialization only with others of the same belief. Even though the rawtarian way of life may ultimately be the one associated with longer life, it is the most difficult one to follow, mainly because of the social challenges and the difficulties in finding healthy, raw food.

24. *What foods are technically "vegan" but are not healthy at all?*

Unhealthy vegan choices are portrayed in some of the meatless burger substitutes, cheese-less cheese substitutes, and white flour products. Reading the labels on these products will show you that they contain mostly processed foods or food products. These fake meat or chicken products may be better than meat, for example; however, they may not necessarily be healthy to eat. Similarly, processed foods such as potato chips, pretzels, candy, and most deserts are a source of wasted calories. Fried foods, like French fries, deep-fried vegetables, and donuts are certainly not healthy. Additionally, sugar content should be taken into consideration in the choice of food to eat, as well as the content of preservatives and other chemical additives.

25. *Can you have a normal social life while being on a healthy diet?*

Eating well does not preclude a happy productive social life unless you feel awkward with your choice. Seemingly when one begins to live affirmatively, they may evangelically want "to convert the masses," often stating that they are trying to help others. In reality, they are actually trying to rally the troops to make their own life easier. Inversely, when you put the healthier food in front of those who feel guilty for eating unhealthily, they are prone to attack and make fun of you. Our best advice is to completely embrace the new cuisine that will fuel a better and longer future and do not try to convince others that they should follow suit. Example is the best teacher. When others criticize you, do not be so thin-skinned and laugh it off increasing your empathy for their struggle. Your job is to do what is best for you and not to be awkward in the process.

26. ***What about entertaining in your home?***

Consciously considering the family and friends whom you bring into your home will determine whether you or they will feel comfortable. Maintaining a plant-based household is not difficult. Many recipe books, websites, and magazines at the checkout line in a supermarket are available to help you prepare interesting meals. Even though some of your friends may not eat the plant-based choices that you offer them, you may be surprised with what they choose. On the other hand, as a host or hostess, be sensitive to people's level of food radar. If you invite heavy meat eaters, it would not be wise to offer them only a salad. You may want to present meat, hamburger, fish, or chicken substitutes. You might not indulge in chips, but you might want to put out healthy varieties of appetizers. Dips are readily available that replace sour cream with tasty substitutes. You might also offer guacamole or one of the many diverse types of hummus. Beverages can be found that are tasty and familiar enough for your guests. To us it is our responsibility to lovingly support those people who we invite into our abode. Entertaining in a plant-based way can become very easy.

27. ***How should you handle yourself when you are asked to go out with friends for a "couple of drinks"?***

It has become clear that many people require alcohol to feel themselves— to feel loose, semi-authentic, uninhibited, albeit only for a brief period. As you mature into a lifestyle that is harmonious with health, your joy factor will rise that is most often followed by greater humor. Many scientific studies emphasize how intestinal bacteria are the most important factors in creating happy heads and socially graceful people. You can order bottled water with lemons as one example, and, if you are in a more enlightened establishment, they might offer herbal teas, non-sugar lemonades, or organic soda choices. Best of all is when the restaurant will make raw vegetable juices for you. There is always a way to manage once you truly manage your own life correctly. Consuming alcohol is not the only way to relax. The same can be said for drugs, whether they be prescription drugs, over-the-counter drugs, or even street drugs. Our culture often revolves around taking drugs, which has to have long-term effects, many of which are not even known.

28. *Is eating breakfast essential? If so, what should you eat? How do you manage a "power breakfast meeting" when bacon, eggs, pancakes, and pastries are all that are available?*

The common conception of breakfast being "the most important meal of the day" may not be true. This concept first was developed in the 1960s when the Baby Boomers were all growing up and is attributed to a famous American nutritionist, Adelle Davis. She is often quoted as saying that to keep fit and avoid obesity, one should "eat breakfast like a king, lunch like a prince, and dinner like a pauper." The reasoning behind that statement is based on the concept that overnight fasting is broken by the consumption of glucose in the food we eat for breakfast, along with the other nutrients contained in the food. It could also be that eating early in the morning keeps your appetite under control for the rest of the day. Unfortunately for some people, that breakfast consists of a donut, pastry, or bagel on the run out the door to work or consumed in the car.

An article written by Lindsey DeSoto and published online (https://www.medicalnewstoday.com/articles/is-breakfast-really-the-most-important-meal-of-the-day) discusses this issue.

Around 15% of people in the United States are estimated to regularly skip breakfast, but many still believe it to be the most important meal of the day (Buckner *et al.*, 2016). Breakfast provides the body with important nutrients to start the day feeling energized and nourished. Many also believe that it can promote weight loss. If one can obtain all the necessary nutrients from food eaten throughout the rest of the day, is there any reason to mandate breakfast? Some people who forgo breakfast consume food-based supplements that may nourish the body rather than consuming food itself.

DeSoto (2022) first looked at the meta-analysis of 14 observational studies from Zhi-hui *et al.* (2021). This study suggested that eating breakfast daily benefits the cardiometabolism to a great extent, reducing the risk of cardiovascular disease, type 2 diabetes, obesity, hypertension, strokes, metabolic syndrome, and overall cardiovascular mortality. This particular group of studies can only suggest that those who eat breakfast are more likely to have a reduced risk for the cardiovascular and metabolic diseases mentioned above. It cannot prove that breakfast is what is causing it. The authors did suggest that skipping breakfast once a week may greatly reduce the benefits of cardiometabolism. This was an observational study, not a double-blind, controlled study. There was also a suggestion that people who skipped breakfast might be missing folic acid, calcium, iron, Vitamin A, and Vitamins B1, B2, B3, C, and D, although there was no objective proof of that.

Around the year 2020, the concept of "intermittent fasting" first became popular, although many people had practiced that concept for years before. This concept is defined differently, by different people, and is almost always individualized by each person to their needs. Some people will undergo a total fast from food for 2 to 3 days per week or every other day. Some people will eat normally for 5 days per week, but radically reduce their caloric intake to fewer than 600 calories per day for the other 2 days. The most commonly used "intermittent fast" is sometimes called the "16:8" in which a person eats only during 8 hours of the day and fasts for the other 16 hours. A researcher at Harvard University, Dr. David Sinclair, has stated that there are four major factors that impact longevity (Sinclair, 2019):

- Calorie restriction
- Food quality
- Exercise
- Cold exposure

His concept is based on preparing our biological survival systems for when we need them the most. That might be why calorie restriction, choice of food, and regular, intense exercise may be the most important.

The concept of intermittent and low-level stress is important. If you do not allow a time for recovery, then there will be limited or no benefit. Think about fasting all the time. Do you know what that is called? It's called "starvation." Think about cold exposure. Intermittent cold exposure activates brown adipose tissue that burns calories to keep you warmer. Too much cold exposure leads to frostbite and tissue damage. When you exercise, you break down muscle and stress joints and ligaments. Almost all the gains come during recovery when your body's DNA are in recovery mode and can transcribe proteins that lead to not only muscle recovery but also muscle growth. The same may be true for emotional stress. We have all seen, or even experienced, the destruction that goes along with chronic stress from a terrible job, family issues, or money woes. Those constant (not intermittent) stressors lead to the breakdown of the human mind, body, and spirit. Low-level stress typically aids in focus and concentration.

Is there any science to support this? A recent study of intermittent fasting was published by Wilkinson *et al.* (2020). They studied a group of people who had metabolic syndrome (a condition associated with hypertension, type 2 diabetes, elevated cholesterol, obesity, and insulin resistance) and who were already on blood pressure and cholesterol medications. The researchers had them eat for only 10 hours a day (fasting for 14 hours a day). The subjects could pick whatever times of the day to eat so long as it was continuous. Within 3 months, the subjects lost weight, lost fat, decreased their waist circumference, lowered their blood pressures, lowered their bad cholesterol levels (LDL), lowered their hemoglobin A1C levels (a measure of diabetic control), and slightly increased their sleep length. What was most impressive about this study is that they did not alter the quality of their diets. They were asked to keep eating the same things they typically ate. They also were not started on any type of new exercise program. The only difference is when they ate! Remember that intermittent fasting is a method of calorie restriction. The subjects in this study ate about 10% less food than they did before the study. If you stuff the same amount of food in during a shorter time interval, it is very unlikely that you will get any of the benefits mentioned above!

The authors also suggested that the easiest way to fast is to fast while you sleep. Even when you sleep, you are burning calories. The more you sleep, the longer you are fasting, and the more calories you are burning! Based on that concept alone, we should all want to sleep more, but do we? About one-third of Americans do not get enough sleep. A good sleep duration is 6 to 9 hours. Less sleep is associated with increased cardiovascular events and death. Many people observe in themselves that if they are up longer, they snack more, especially before going to bed. Unfortunately, eating before going to sleep is often associated with poor sleep, which is counterproductive to healthy living.

Theoretically, fasting increases the production of a hormone called *leptin*, which is a naturally occurring anti-hunger hormone that may signal our brains not to be hungry.

So, the concept of intermittent fasting is an interesting one to consider. It might help you lose weight, burn fat, lower your blood sugar (if you have type 2 diabetes), lower your blood pressure (if you have hypertension), and improve your cholesterol, if that is a problem for you. It might even help you live longer if you can control those risk factors.

Again, the studies are only observational, not evidence based. It is now up to you to choose between the "traditional" breakfast and intermittent fasting. Whichever eating style you choose, do NOT eat bacon, eggs, pancakes, and pastries for breakfast. THAT makes no sense. For some, fruit (alone) may be an option or even a vegetable salad with sprouts may be another viable option.

This intermittent fasting is so popular that if you are invited to a "power breakfast" meeting (unlikely for most of us who are retired), and it is not time for you to eat on your personal schedule, just tell the others at the meeting, "My doctor told me to eat this way. It will improve my life span." They may actually take you seriously!

As with all our suggestions, since there are no research-based studies about eating or not eating breakfast, the choice is again up to you. Maybe now you have enough information to make that choice for yourself.

The last comment is about hunger. People are afraid if they fast or even miss a meal, they will feel "hungry," so they would never consider fasting. Hunger, unfortunately, is a very subjective feeling. Some people eat because they are tired, stressed, anxious, or upset, rather than truly lacking in body nourishment. Some people attribute that feeling to low blood sugar levels, but that observation has never been studied in a scientific way. The concept of "hunger" seems to improve when one is on an intermittent fasting program.

29. What about "gluten-free" foods, like pasta? Are they acceptable to eat?

Originally, wheat was small in size, dark in color, and high in protein, up to 36% by weight. Over the years, humans began to consume wheat and wheat products. In fact, wheat became known as the "Staff of Life." As a marked need appeared to supply more and more wheat, agricultural engineers began to modify the nutritional structure of wheat. Part of the wheat contains proteins that are called "gluten." Gluten helps foods maintain their shape, acting as a glue that holds food together. This gluten can also be found in wheatberries, semolina, spelt, farina, farro, graham, kamut, as well as rye, barley, and triticale. In fact, gluten works so well as a binding agent to hold processed foods together and give them shape, that gluten can be extracted, concentrated, and added to food and other products to add protein, texture, and even flavor.

So, what is the problem? Humans have digestive enzymes that help us break down food. Protease is the enzyme that helps our body process proteins, but it struggles to break down gluten. Undigested gluten makes its way to the small intestine. Most people can manage the undigested gluten without problems. In some people, however, gluten can trigger a severe autoimmune response or other unpleasant symptoms.

The autoimmune response to gluten is called "celiac disease," which can damage the small intestine. Some people who do not have celiac disease still seem to feel sick after eating foods that contain gluten, with bloating, diarrhea, headaches, or skin rashes. This could be a reaction to poorly digested carbohydrates, not just gluten. These carbs ferment in your intestines. People with sensitive guts may experience discomfort from that fermentation, not necessarily from gluten. Those folks do not have celiac disease.

Some confusion exists about gluten being an evil food. Gluten is not inherently bad for most people. Humans have consumed gluten for as long as people have been making bread. For centuries, foods with gluten have been providing people with protein, soluble fiber, and nutrients. Gluten, especially gluten found in whole grains, is not bad for healthy people whose bodies can tolerate it. However, grains like wheat are often stripped down to make processed foods such as snack crackers and potato chips. These refined products have very little resemblance to the actual wheat plant, which is highly nutritious. They tend to contain things like white rice flour and starches, but not whole grains.

Gluten can be harmful to some people with the following health issues:

- Celiac disease (an autoimmune disease that causes damage to the small intestine in people who consume gluten).
- Non-celiac gluten sensitivity (also called "gluten intolerance") (a gastrointestinal irritation caused by gluten in people who do not have celiac disease. Some symptoms can include headaches, bloating, runny nose, and joint pain. It could possibly cause memory loss in some people).
- Wheat allergy (an allergy to wheat, but not to all grains or to gluten itself).
- Gluten ataxia (a very rare neurological disorder that causes your body to attack parts of your brain in response to gluten).

For those people who want to consume foods that might be considered like those that contain gluten, it is quite easy to find gluten-free pasta (made from lentils, quinoa, mung beans, rice, and peas), which is quite tasty and readily available. Gluten-free pizza in which the crust is made from cauliflower is also available in some restaurants and in the frozen food section of a grocery store. In fact, more and more products in grocery stores contain the label "gluten-free" as do menu choices in some restaurants. Years ago, having gluten intolerance or even celiac disease was a curse, but now it is so commonplace that one can live a perfectly normal life without the inconvenience of shopping or eating out at certain places.

30. *Which vegetables and fruits should never be eaten unless they are organic?*
A. Nonorganic foods are contaminated, so to speak, with pesticides, herbicides, and fertilizers. Could those be detrimental to your health?

Not only are pesticides dangerous to the environment, but they may also be hazardous to a person's health. Pesticides are stored in your colon, where they slowly but surely poison the body. You may not realize this, but when you are eating a nonorganic apple, you are also eating over 30 different pesticides that have been sprayed on the apple. Even if you wash a piece of fruit, such as an apple, many pesticides may linger on it, and they could have seeped into the fruit or vegetable. All this information can be found on the website of the EPA.

After countless studies, pesticides have been linked to cancer, Alzheimer's disease, maybe even ADHD and birth defects. Pesticides also have the potential to harm the nervous system, the reproductive system, and even the endocrine system. Pesticides can even be very harmful to fetuses because the chemicals can pass from the mother during pregnancy or if a woman nurses her child. Although one piece of contaminated fruit will not kill you, pesticide contamination can build up in your body and might be detrimental to your health over the years. That is why eating as much organic food as possible is the only way to prevent those potential problems.

What if you cannot find organic, pesticide-free foods? An organization called the EWG publishes each year something that is often quoted, called the "Dirty Dozen" and the "Clean Fifteen." They state that you should only consume organic, pesticide-free foods, but if you cannot find those foods, there are certain fruits and vegetables that you should avoid at all costs.

These are called "**The Dirty Dozen**." Here they are for 2022:

1. Strawberries
2. Spinach
3. Kale
4. Nectarines
5. Apples
6. Grapes
7. Bell & hot peppers
8. Cherries
9. Peaches
10. Pears
11. Celery
12. Tomatoes

On the other end of the spectrum, they have identified fewer pesticides on the following set of fruits and vegetables, which they call their **"Clean Fifteen"**:

1. Avocados
2. Sweet Corn
3. Pineapple
4. Onions
5. Papaya
6. Frozen Sweet Peas
7. Asparagus
8. Honeydew melon
9. Kiwi
10. Cabbage
11. Mushrooms
12. Cantaloupe
13. Mangoes
14. Watermelon
15. Sweet potatoes

By avoiding contaminated foods, you have the maximum chance to stay healthy. Again, we cannot affirmatively state that eating this way will make you live longer, but you will optimize your health in that way which might contribute to longevity.

31. *What percentage of your diet should be cooked and what percentage uncooked?*

When a person has a disease like cancer, multiple sclerosis, and maybe Parkinson's disease, there are anecdotal and observational studies suggesting that adhering to a raw, organic plant-based diet might help prolong life. This is not saying that you should stop conventional medical advice but view the diet as a complement to medical care. In those situations, it makes total sense to follow the raw food diet intensely. Once you have come into recovery or once you have adjusted to that lifestyle as you work on yourself, whether to lose weight, to feel better, to sleep better, and maybe to manage stress better—all of which just might be possible on a raw, plant-based diet, you might feel just as well on a diet that is 75% raw and 25% cooked. Some laboratory studies have shown that activity of immune cells was better on a raw food diet, but not much different on a 75:25 diet. Again, we are not saying that being on a raw food diet has been proven to make you live longer, but it does make you healthier and feel better. Healthy people seem to live longer. We are not saying you must be 100% raw, but rather you should make as many choices of raw, uncooked foods as possible.

32. What should you do when you go on a vacation, including going on a cruise?

Planning seems like a unique concept in the haphazard world we all live in. Yet it makes smooth travels appear. If you are determined to do so, you will never miss a beat when it comes to consistent healthy food selections and ongoing exercise. PRIORITY, PRIORITY! PRIORITY! When you make yourself important enough to do the right thing, everything becomes second nature. Today's Internet world has amplified the ease. Many websites and search engines will direct you to where the closest health restaurants or gyms are. You might even find yourself in many far lands that you would not expect offer healthy choices. Yet, with the right attitude and determination, you will never have any problem at any time eating well and taking care of yourself.

Cruises happen to be one of the best vacations for relaxation. Years ago, requesting a vegetarian meal plan meant you were served spaghetti and tomato sauce or eggplant parmesan, with the same entrees offered each night. Then vegie-burgers became available. No one else who sat at your table would ever want what you were served for dinner. Things have changed. Now, a phone call to the cruise line will ensure that you have a relatively healthy (probably not organic) dinner with many choices of options that change each day. By the end of the cruise, many of the other passengers at your table might even request to have what you are being served. Plant-based eating is no longer obscure. In fact, it is the growing norm for the global population. When young people are polled, they are either vegan, partially vegan, or are aspiring to be vegan in over half of the population. In certain countries like Israel, England, and even the western part of the United States, plant-based foods are widely available in a majority of supermarkets, restaurants, and fast-food chains. Countries like Poland and even the United Nations have stated "For human and planetary survival, the future will include plant-based fare."

33. *What should you do when you are flying on an airplane and the flight attendant brings you drinks and snacks?*

Dietitians or food planners who create low-cost food offerings on planes seemingly miss the part in their education where "Food Is Medicine." When traveling, it is best to eat lightly and drink plenty of pure fluids before boarding the plane. On longer trips, like cross-country or international travel, some people advise only to drink fluids on such flights. Some people also are concerned about the low-level radiation in the sky when you fly. Drinking fluids is probably the only thing that you can do to minimize effects from air travel. Again, it is nothing to worry about if you travel occasionally around the world. According to the CDC in 2015, the exposure to low-level radiation is less than that received with a chest x-ray. More serious are the snacks that the airlines offer to their passengers. There is nothing healthy about any of them, and it is best to say no to the flight attendant who offers you a choice.

34. *What do you tell people who constantly ask you, "Why are you not having protein with your meal?"*

Ironically, all proteins we eat originate from plants. For this reason, when you think about it, why are some people consuming animal protein that was derived from plants in the first place? There are many professional athletes who realized early in their careers, like Mohammad Ali, Venus and Serena Williams, as well as some top bodybuilders, that consuming protein does not always mean eating meat, chicken, and fish.

In the early 20th century, the meat and dairy industries connived to create scare tactics that would work best to promote their products. Without scientific support, the promoters worked their way into our educational material, creating the façade that we would starve without consumption of animal flesh, and that our bones would disintegrate without consumption of milk. In the 21st century not only have those pieces of "fake news" been debunked but there are endless studies that elimination of those animal products might deliver a longer and healthier life.

As always, we can only present ideas and discuss choices. You have the right to make your own choice as to what works for you.

35. *How will you get enough Vitamin B12? Are any other vitamins or minerals missing if you give up eating animal products?*

According to the Mayo Clinic, Vitamin B12 (also called "cobalamin") plays an essential role in red blood cell formation, cell metabolism, nerve function, and the production of DNA. Food sources of B12 include meat, poultry, fish, and daily products. B12 is also added to some foods, including fortified breakfast cereals, and is available as an oral supplement. Vitamin B12 injections or even nasal spray might be prescribed to treat B_{12} deficiency. Left untreated, a Vitamin B12 deficiency can lead to anemia, fatigue, muscle weakness, intestinal problems, nerve damage, and mood disturbances.

Vitamin B12 deficiency is not common in the United States. Older adults and people with digestive tract conditions that affect absorption of nutrients also are susceptible to Vitamin B12 deficiency.

Over the years, there have developed several myths about B12 and its use for nonspecific symptoms. At one time, researchers believed that taking B12, along with folic acid (B9) and Vitamin B6, might prevent heart disease by reducing the levels of an amino acid called homocysteine. However, subsequent studies refuted that. Currently, there is no evidence that taking B12 alone or in combination with the other vitamins mentioned above will do anything to prevent cardiovascular disease.

Vitamin B12 deficiency is associated with dementia, but there is no evidence that taking supplemental B12, without known B12 deficiency, will treat or prevent dementia. It will not Improve athletic performance or improve nonspecific symptoms (tiredness, fatigue, muscle aches). Patients have been asking their health care providers to make them feel better with B12 supplements, injections, or infusions. There are no data to support that.

If it is not clear whether you have B12 deficiency, you can ask your health care provider to order a specific blood test to measure your B12 concentration. The results might guide you into whether you need supplementation. If you suffer from a rare disease called "Pernicious Anemia," your body does not have the ability to absorb B12 no matter what the source. You will need monthly injections of B12. Oral replacement of B12 will not work as the B12 will not be absorbed.

If you do not have Pernicious Anemia and feel you still need B12, you can take B12 orally.

B12 is thought to be made by bacteria in the soil and absorbed by plants. Animals, like cows and sheep, have B12 because they eat plants. Humans seem to need about 2.4 mcg to 2.8 mcg of B12 daily. Older people may have some difficulty with B12 absorption as do some people with prior surgery on their digestive tracts.

If you are a pure vegan (no meat, dairy, eggs), you will need B12 supplements. You can empirically take Vitamin B12 supplements, or you can measure your level of B12 in your blood first and then decide if you need to take supplements. It is not known if you can get enough B12 by eating a piece of fish or chicken once a month or even once a week. Always be safe, since toxicity from too much B12 is quite minimal.

The best form of B12 to take is a plant-based form of B12 supplements which are readily available.

36. Can you stay on a plant-based program forever? Are there any published scientific studies to confirm that plant-based is the way to go?
As in all dietary programs, there are no research-based programs using age- and gender-matched subjects who have been followed for many years. It is an impossible task, so all we have are observational studies. In his book *The China Study*, Campbell and Campbell (2006) discussed the high frequency of cancer, heart disease, and diabetes in people who consumed large amounts of animal products, including dairy and eggs. There are many similar studies, but no prospective ones. A dietitian at Cleveland Clinic, Julie Zumpano, wrote in her book, *What You Should Know about Plant-Based Diets—Cleveland Clinic*, that research reflects that following a plant-based diet has significant health benefits as long as you do it correctly. If followed properly, a whole-food, plant-based diet limits the use of oils, added sugars, and processed foods, leaving only whole foods to provide nutrition. This maximizes nutrient intake and virtually eliminates foods that can lead to poor health outcomes. These diets are low in saturated fat, free of cholesterol, and rich in fiber, vitamins, minerals, and antioxidants.

Following a plant-based diet means saying goodbye to all animal products, which is easier said than done for many people. It requires knowledge, information, and practice, including understanding food choices, knowledge of where to obtain protein, and which foods should be chosen, even if you are not used to eating them.

37. Tell us about "food combining." Is it essential? Will you feel better doing it and worse if you do not?
Food combining is a philosophy of eating that has been around since ancient times, but it has become popular in recent years. Proponents of food-combining diets believe that improper food combinations can lead to disease, toxin buildup, and digestive issues. They also believe that

proper combinations can help relieve these problems. But is there any truth to these claims?

Food combining is a concept based on the idea that certain foods pair well, while others do not. All members of the animal kingdom eat one thing at a time. This "mono diet" works for them. Lions do not eat one catch, then some grass, then something sweet before they go to sleep. Humans have adapted the practice of mixing or combining different foods with each meal. For example, what steak restaurant does not serve steak and potatoes? This concept can be traced back to the ancient Ayurvedic medicine of India, but the concept became popular in the 1800s. In simplicity, food-combining diets assign certain foods to different groups. These are usually broken down into carbohydrates (starches), fruits (including sweet fruits, acidic fruits, and melons), vegetables, proteins, and fats. Some of these diet plans classify foods as acidic, alkaline, or neutral.

The rules of proper food combining vary between individuals, but include the following:

- Eat fruit only on an empty stomach, especially melons.
- Avoid combining starches and proteins.
- Avoid combining starches with acidic foods.
- Avoid combing distinct types of proteins.
- If you consume dairy products, only do so on an empty stomach.
- Protein should not be mixed with fat.
- Fruits and vegetables should be eaten separately.

The theory behind this style of eating is that foods are digested at different rates. When one eats fast-digesting food with slow-digesting food, there may be issues in the digestive system, leading to problems with adequate digestion of both. In addition, different foods require different digestive enzymes which work differently depending on what food needs to be digested. The end-result is that improper food combining might lead to digestive symptoms and maybe disease.

Unfortunately, there are no scientific studies to confirm whether this type of eating has any long- or short-term benefits. If this makes sense to you, try it for a while, maybe even in a residential program. If you feel better, then continue. We chose to include this lifestyle as an option for some people to consider. There are many books and articles written on this subject.

38. *Should you start a plant-based diet all at once or gradually ease into it?*

This question can only be answered with another question. Are you one who is wise enough to know that your food choices are counterproductive to your well-being and longevity or are you one who realizes your past food choices are what created your disorders and premature aging? The first group without serious diagnosis can casually move into an approved diet and lifestyle. You may say in one year I will be 50% there and in two years I will be 100% there.

Those who are facing illnesses, serious immobility, and/or chronic pain do not have the luxury to move slowly. These individuals need to jump into the cold water and learn how to swim. Attending a residential comprehensive guided life transformation program has provided thousands a fruitful starting point for their new lifestyle. Others will read, watch programs on the Internet, join health-minded organizations, or find friends who share their mindset. Understanding that what you do every single day with your attitude, food, exercise, and relationships determines your level of health and happiness should inspire you to get to where you need to be as soon as you possibly can. Once you immerse yourself into healing and wellness, it becomes ever increasingly easier to move forward in a graceful and effective manner.

39. *Are there any benefits from the use of a residential program to get started?*

Residential programs, where you leave your normal home environment and stay in a hotel-like room and are fed a diet totally appropriate to your body's needs, are frequently the best way to get started on any life-changing effort. Often people who need to make such a change will have had ample opportunities to do so on their own, like trying to lose weight or beginning an exercise program, but they just don't. It is often the obligations of day-to-day life that make that type of commitment very difficult to make. Going to a residential program removes a person from a "normal" routine, removes much of the external stress, and gives a chance to live the life that one is trying to achieve. Therefore, it seems logical that going away to a facility is the best way to get started. There are many programs around, but each person needs to find the program that matches her or his goals. Staying for a "long weekend" might be a start, but it is not recommended. We feel that to make a major change one needs 30 days. Most people cannot afford to take off 4 weeks, but usually 3 weeks or 2 weeks can be achieved easily. Just think about going on a cruise. A cruise is often 2 or 3 weeks in duration. Yet, when you leave the cruise ship at the end, you often feel terrible. You overeat, overdrink, and only exercise by walking around the ports. Going to a residential program where only organic, healthy food is served, enrolling in group and individual exercise programs that are readily available, and joining classes offered all day in life-changing ideas are a wonderful way to start. At the end of the 2 or 3 weeks, you feel great, and, for those of you who need to lose weight, you may happen to lose 10 to 15 pounds. Recidivism is always a problem when you change lifestyles out of choice, rather than necessity. For most people, expect that you will need a "refresher" from time to time. If you can hold out 6 months, going back to the program for 1 week every 6 months is a real option. When you find a program that you like, you trust, you learn from and works for you, keep going back.

40. *What if you "eat healthy" 80% of the time, indulging in a steak or a piece of broiled fish "once in a while"?*

That is an impossible question to answer. There has never been, nor will there ever be, a research study to answer that question. All we can recommend is that all your dietary suggestions should make sense, either based on scientific studies or extensive personal observations. You must be the one who decides how strictly you want to adhere to a healthy lifestyle and what deviations will you allow yourself to take. It seems reasonable, but certainly not proved, that the stricter you are with your eating, the better the chance you will have to stay healthy for many years.

41. *I am 76 years old and want to live to 120. Is it too late for me to have any beneficial effects by changing my diet?*

Not at all. A study by Lasheras *et al.* (2000) looked at people over 65 who were able to change their diets to those of Mediterranean diets. They found increased longevity in their subjects. So, you are never too old to eat healthy.

CHAPTER
2

Exercise

Suppose a pharmaceutical company discovered a new drug that helps you get fit, reduces your body weight, improves your balance, and lowers your risk for many diseases, such as high blood pressure, diabetes, and heart disease, and is readily available. You do have to take it once a day, maybe three times each week, and it is free! Who would turn that down, right?

Welcome to the world of *exercise*. Exercise is anti-inflammatory, boosts mood, improves sleep, improves cognitive function, reduces memory loss, improves digestion, and improves the immune system, but does it make you live longer?

Many scientific studies have been published over the past 20 years looking at exercise intervention for older adults in reducing the chance of developing or reducing the severity of atherosclerotic heart disease, improving blood sugar levels in patients with type 2 diabetes, including reducing or withdrawing patients from medications, controlling blood pressure, improving blood cholesterol levels, and recently found to delay the progression of Parkinson's disease symptoms. A study from Brigham Young University (2017), published in *Preventive Medicine*, showed that high levels of physical activity (PA) equated to a nine-year biological aging advantage. They looked at the extent to which physical activity accounts for differences in leukocyte telomere length (LTL) in a large random sample of U.S. adults and to assess the extent to which multiple demographic and lifestyle covariates affect the relationship between PA and LTL. Those researchers found that the telomeres, the end caps on chromosomes that shorten with age, were longer in people who were active compared to those who were inactive.

A meta-analysis (Watts, 2022) showed that moderately active women had a 24% lower risk of death, and the most active women had a 31% lower risk of death. The corresponding results for men were 19% and 24%. Among vigorously physically active, however, the risk of sudden cardiac death is increased during episodic physical activity. Slowly increasing the levels of habitual physical activity was associated with progressively lower relative risks of myocardial infarction during episodic vigorous physical activity.

A study from the Cleveland Clinic (Harb *et al.*, 2019) looked at over 120,000 patients, from ages 18 to 80. The study found that cardiorespiratory fitness is inversely associated with long-term mortality with no observed upper limit of benefit. Extremely high aerobic fitness was associated with marked benefit in older patients.

Another meta-analysis (Caliebe *et al.*, 2010) looked at life expectancy in physically active and inactive individuals. They found that regular physical activity reduced the risk of and/or improved many diseases and conditions, including hypertension, type 2 diabetes, dyslipidemia, obesity, coronary heart disease, chronic heart failure, and chronic obstructive pulmonary disease. In addition, the risks of colon, breast, and, possibly, endometrial, lung, and pancreatic cancer were reduced. All-cause mortality decreased by about 30–35% in physically active, as compared to inactive, subjects. They went on to speculate that this significant increase in longevity might be related to reduction of triglyceride and apolipoprotein B (ApoB) concentrations, increase of high-density lipoproteins and tissue plasminogen activator activity, and reduction of coronary artery calcium resulting in reduced risks of vascular diseases, which carry the strongest mortality risk. In addition, regular physical activity increases the endurance of cells and tissues to oxidative stress, vascularization, and energy metabolism. Physical exercise may also reduce the incidence of dementia.

Intense exercise seems to be an integral part of the management of Parkinson's disease because physical activity has been shown to delay the deterioration of motor functions and to prolong functional independence (*New England Journal of Medicine*, 1961; *Neurology*, 2022).

Osteoporosis is characterized by the loss of calcium in a person's bones, which makes them more likely to fracture. Weight-bearing exercising regularly reduces the rate of bone loss and conserves bone tissue, lowering the risk of fractures. Exercise also helps reduce the risk of falling.

As was noted in our introduction, despite advances in medicine, health care, and social conditions, longer life expectancy is not necessarily matched with increased health. Engagement in exercise has multiple health benefits and can slow some of the negative effects of aging. Exercise improves physiological outcomes in older people who have gone through long periods of sedentary lifestyle, nonagenarians, and older individuals with frailty or *osteopenia* (thin bones). Exercise is defined as "planned, structured, and repetitive physical activity."

In addition, exercise makes you feel good, look good, have more confidence, be more relaxed, and live longer.

So, let's get "moving!"

According to the CDC (*Physical Activity Guidelines for Americans*, 2nd edition), in 2018, the percentage of adults aged 18 and over who met the Physical Activity Guidelines for aerobic physical activity was 53.3%. In a different study, nationally, 22.9% of U.S. adults aged 18 to 64 met the guidelines for both aerobic and muscle-strengthening activities during leisure-time physical activity between 2010 and 2015.

The CDC also has set a goal of increasing physical activity among all Americans and has measured progress, at least in part, by examining state-level information on physical activity. Physical activities can be classified as recreational (taking place during leisure time), occupational (taking place during the performance of work, including household tasks), or it can include walking or cycling specifically for transportation or commuting.

Using population-based data from the 2001 National Health Interview Survey, Kruger *et al.* (2007) classified qualified respondents (N = 11,969) according to whether they met the activity criteria used in *Healthy People 2010* goals for leisure-time participation in regular aerobic physical activity, vigorous-intensity aerobic activity, strength-training activity, and flexibility activity. They also classified respondents according to their level of aerobic activity (*i.e.*, inactive, insufficiently active, and regularly active). They estimated that 46.4% of older Americans were engaged in no leisure-time aerobic activity; that 26.1% were regularly active (participated in light-to-moderate-intensity aerobic activities at least 5 days per week for at least 30 minutes or vigorous-intensity activities at least 3 days per week for at least 20 minutes); that 16.2% participated in vigorous-intensity aerobic activities at least 3 days per week for at least 20 minutes; that 13.7% participated in strength-training activities at least 2 days per week; and that 24.5% participated in flexibility activities at least 1 day per week. Among the 26.1% of older Americans who were regularly active, 30.5% engaged in strengthen-training activities at least 2 days per week. Overall, only 8.2% of older Americans met the criteria for both aerobic and strength-training activity. We think you can do better, especially if you want to live long.

According to Dr. Lauren Elson, writing in the *Harvard Health Blog*, June 25, 2019 (Elson, 2019) the federal government's Office of Disease Prevention and Health Promotion issued guidelines to follow. Their recommendations range from a high of 3 hours daily for preschool children to 150 minutes per week for adults. Despite those relatively low standards, 80% of the population is not meeting them. Each year in the United States, an estimated 10% of premature deaths and $117 billion in health care costs are associated with inadequate activity. *The Physical Activity Guidelines for Americans*, 2nd edition (https:// health.gov/our-work/nutrition-physical-activity/physical-activity-guidelines/

current-guidelines/top-10-things-know) state that adults need at least 150–300 minutes of moderate-intensity aerobic activity, like brisk walking or fast dancing each week, or they need 75 minutes of vigorous-intensity activity, such as hiking, jogging, or running. Adults also need muscle-strengthening activity, like lifting weights or doing pushups, at least 2 days each week. She also recommends activities to improve balance, such as standing on one foot about 3 days a week.

Obviously, the benefits of physical activity occur throughout life and are essential for healthy aging. Baby Boomers can gain substantial health benefits from regular physical activity. Even though a large percentage of us do no regular exercise, it is never too late. By doing so, it will become easier to perform activities of daily living, such as bathing, toileting, dressing, getting into and out of bed or a chair, and even walking around the house. Physically active adults are less likely to experience falls, and if they do fall, are less likely to be seriously injured. Physical activity can also preserve physical function and mobility, which may help people retain their independence from chronic care. It is well known that our generation or the generation older than us is the least physically active of any age group. In fact, most very old people (those over 85) spend a sizable portion of their day being sedentary.

What may be some reasons for that? Possibly, a person has underlying medical problems, such as heart disease, poor circulation, or even balance problems, any of which can cause that person to avoid any exercise. Some people, as noted above, have not exercised for years and are so out of shape that they feel nervous at doing any form of exercise. Some people may be so overweight that they are embarrassed in wearing exercise clothes to the gym. Maybe some people do not like to sweat so they avoid any exercise. People who do not exercise always have their own personal reasons for not doing so.

Being physically active is key to preventing and managing some chronic diseases. Some researchers even feel that people who exercise have a lower incidence of dementia, such as Alzheimer's disease. The same is true for a better perception of the quality of life, and reduced anxiety and depression. Completing physical activity with others can provide the socialization that is also a factor in longevity (and will be discussed in Chapter 5). It is very hard to generalize since all adults do experience some type of physical decline with aging, but everyone is totally different in the speed of that loss and the specific issues related.

The U.S. Department of Health and Human Services published the *Physical Activity Guidelines for Americans,* 2nd edition in 2018. Included are guidelines that are applicable to Baby Boomers.

Key Guidelines for Older Adults (Source: Physical Activity Guidelines for Americans, 2nd ed.)

These guidelines are the same for all adults, including older adults:

- Adults should move more and sit less throughout the day. Some physical activity is better than none. Adults who sit less and do any amount of moderate-to-vigorous physical activity gain some health benefits.
- For substantial health benefits, adults should do at least 150 minutes (2 hours and 30 minutes) to 300 minutes (5 hours) a week of moderate-intensity, or 75 minutes (1 hour and 15 minutes) to 150 minutes (2 hours and 30 minutes) a week of vigorous-intensity aerobic physical activity, or an equivalent combination of moderate- and vigorous-intensity aerobic activity. Preferably, aerobic activity should be spread through the week.
- Additional health benefits are gained by engaging in physical activity beyond the equivalent of 300 minutes (5 hours) of moderate-intensity physical activity a week.
- Adults should also do muscle-strengthening activities of moderate or greater intensity and that involve all major muscle groups on 2 or more days a week, as these activities provide additional health benefits.

Guidelines just for older adults:

- As part of their weekly physical activity, older adults should do multicomponent physical activity that includes balance training as well as aerobic and muscle-strengthening activities.
- Older adults should determine their level of effort for physical activity relative to their level of fitness.
- Older adults with chronic conditions should understand whether and how their conditions affect their ability to do regular physical activity safely.
- When older adult cannot do 150 minutes of moderate-intensity aerobic activity a week because of chronic conditions, they should be as physically active as their abilities and conditions allow.

The key guidelines for older adults focus mainly on specific types of activities:

- Aerobic
- Flexibility
- Muscle-strengthening
- Balance

In addition, the guidelines emphasize the importance of multicomponent physical activity that includes balance training along with aerobic and muscle-strengthening activity.

Aerobic Activity

These activities, also called "endurance" or "cardio" activities, are physical activities in which people move their large muscles in a rhythmic manner for sustained periods of time.

The federal guidelines include the following:

- Brisk walking
- Jogging
- Biking
- Dancing
- Swimming
- Cycling

We realize that people need more choices, so we have organized the activities listed below as indoor or outdoor. Outdoor activities can be done only during warmer weather, unless you live in Florida, California, or places with warm weather, so we have included many other activities to choose from:

Indoors:

At home
Treadmill
Stationary bicycle
Elliptical machine
Traditional calisthenics

In a pool
Walking
Swimming
Water aerobics class
Underwater treadmill

In the gym
Treadmill
Elliptical machine
Stair climber
Recumbent bike
Stationary bike
Spinning class
Peloton bike
Rowing machine
Aerobic exercise class
Pilates/Yoga

Outdoors:

Walking	Snowshoe walking
Brisk walking	Cross-country skiing
Jogging	Rollerblading
Cycling (2- or 3-wheel bike)	Yard work
Skiing	Tennis (singles is better than doubles)
Snowboarding	Pickle ball

How much minimal total activity should a Baby Boomer strive for?

The same CDC guidelines recommend at least 150 minutes of moderate-intensity physical activity each week. Alternatively, this can be satisfied with vigorous-intensity activity at 75 to 150 minutes each week. A greater amount of physical activity results in a reduced risk of age-related loss of function and reduced risk of physical function limitations. This type of activity should be spread throughout the week. Research studies show that activity performed on at least 3 days a week produces health benefits. Spreading it out might also help to reduce the risk of injury and prevent excessive fatigue.

How intense is "intense"?

This depends upon how fit you are. If a person usually rides a bicycle at 12 miles per hour for 1 hour, she or he feels comfortable, and the heart rate stays close to her or his resting rate. If a person pushes herself or himself to 18 miles per hour, the heart rate increases, as does the breathing rate. Professional cyclists in competition often average 26 miles per hour riding uphill! Riding at 15 miles per hour, they would not even break a sweat.

The same guidelines define "absolute intensity" as the amount of energy expended during the activity without considering a person's cardiorespiratory fitness. The energy expenditure of light-intensity activity, for example, is 1.6 to 2.9 times the amount of energy expended when a person is at rest. Moderate-intensity activities expend 3.0 to 5.9 times the amount of energy expended at rest, while the energy expenditure of vigorous-intensity activities is 6.0 times the energy expended at rest.

"Relative intensity" refers to the level of effort required to perform an activity. The example we gave a few paragraphs above about cyclists is a typical example. Less fit people generally require a higher level of effort than more fit people to perform the same activity. The relative intensity of aerobic activity is related to a person's level of cardiorespiratory fitness.

A well-accepted rule of thumb is that a healthy person can calculate her or his maximum heart rate by using the formula of 220 minus the person's age in years. Intense exercise, therefore, means exercising at 60–80% of that maximum rate. For example, if a person is 70 years old, 220 − 70 = 150 which is considered the maximum heart rate and 60% of that is 90; 80% of that is 120, so that person should try to sustain a heart rate of 90–120 for the duration of the activity. Scientists have found that some people cannot get their heart rates up to the maximum as defined by the formula because of underlying intrinsic heart problems associated with aging. In addition, other people take heart or blood pressure–lowering medications, which also can prevent achieving maximum heart rate. However, the formula above will work fine for most people. Another way to reach the rate needed for intensive exercise is called the "perceived level of intensity." If you walk with another person and can carry on a conversation, the exercise is great, but it is not considered intense. If you walk or jog or bike-ride so fast that you can barely speak to your exercise partner, you are exercising in that proper range.

Flexibility (Stretching)

If less than 10% of seniors do enough exercise to meet the CDC's recommendations, even less than that may do sufficient flexibility training or stretching. Nearly everyone over 65 has developed some type of arthritis. Arthritis (also called "degenerative joint disease") is the most common form of arthritis, affecting millions of people worldwide. It occurs when the protective cartilage that cushions the ends of the bones wears down over time. Although arthritis can damage any joint, the disorder most commonly affects joints in your hands, knees, hips, shoulders, and spine. Probably, some people who you know have had joint replacement surgery of their knees, hips, or shoulders and laminectomies or back fusion surgery for severe pain and limitation of movement caused by degenerative arthritis.

Besides anti-inflammatory medications, cortisone injections, and surgery, there are things that can be done. Most seniors are relatively immobile, or if they are active, they often choose just one "event," such as walking. Rarely do they pay attention to other areas of their body, such has shoulders, hips, knees, spine, chest muscles, hamstrings, quadriceps muscles, and abdominal muscles. Stretching properly, usually with the assistance of a class or an individual trainer, can go a long way to improve symptoms of arthritis, increase mobility, improve stiffness, and make a person feel better.

The downside of starting such a program is that seeing results may not come as quickly as seeing results from aerobic activity or weight training. Stretching is a commitment that one makes to improve one's life. It just takes time. The longer it has been (possibly never) since one undertook a stretching program, the longer it will take to start to feel better. Three or four months of this work is not unreasonable.

Where should you start? Many gyms offer stretching classes. Be careful because some of the classes are quite large. At first you may be extremely limited compared to others in the class. It is easy to get discouraged when you compare yourself to others. Keep in mind that no one else really cares how good or how flexible you are. You are doing this for yourself. If you can find and can afford a personal trainer, make sure that the person is used to working with seniors and understands the concept of "gentle stretching," not like something that an athlete needs to do for increased performance.

In the past few years, franchises have been appearing who offer just stretching. This is something to consider if there is such a store in your neighborhood. Many YouTube videos are available for stretching and other downloadable materials to follow.

The last suggestion is that of Yoga. In a later chapter, we will talk about the life extension associated with Yoga and Meditation, but now we are telling you about Yoga as a flexibility exercise. Yoga classes come in all varieties. Many are very intense and are filled with young people in amazing shape and with amazing flexibility. These classes go very fast and are not for you. Look for Yoga Stretch classes, or better yet, Yin Yoga, which has gentle activities, and emphasizes slow movements and sustained positions. It will take you several weeks in the beginning to get used to these classes but keep them up. They last about an hour, and each instructor does the workout differently, which is even better for you. Each instructor and each class will emphasize different muscle groups and different stretches. Your flexibility will improve and just maybe your arthritic pain will improve.

We do not have any data about prolonging life with more flexibility, but you will surely feel much better.

Muscle-Strengthening Activities

Aerobic activities are easy to quantify in terms of duration and intensity of the exercise. Muscle-strengthening activities are vaguer, but equally essential, to maintain health and prevent injury. It is recommended that older adults do muscle-strengthening activities at least twice a week. These activities involve using the legs, hips, chest, back, abdomen, shoulders, and arms. The improvements in muscle are specific to the muscles used in the activity. Examples:

Weightlifting
Working with resistance bands or cords
Pushups, pull-ups, or planks
Stair climbing
Shoveling snow
Carrying heavy loads (*e.g.*, groceries)

There are specific guidelines for the time needed to be spent in muscle-strengthening work. Trainers often recommend sets of repetitions of one exercise for a specific muscle group, like two to three sets, or until muscle fatigue occurs. Some people like to gradually increase the amount of resistance over time as they get stronger. At least when you are first starting out, it is usually simple to develop a routine or program for strength training with a professional. This option is far underutilized. For the majority of Americans, this is the least practiced, and probably the reason why people shy away from ever starting muscle-strengthening exercises.

Balance Activities

As we all age, our balance tends to deteriorate. Notice when you have to stand on one leg to put on a pair of pants. You might be shaky on one side or the other and tend to fall. Therefore, the purpose of balance work is to reduce the risk of injury (such as a fractured hip from a fall). Some of the exercises to consider include:

Walking heel-to-toe
Practicing standing from a sitting position
Using a wobble board

Now for some practical suggestions. As in the previous chapter, these will be addressed in a question-and-answer format.

1. *"I have not exercised since I was in college. Where shall I start? I am 74 years old, have no known medical conditions, and am of near average weight."*

It is not reasonable to expect that suddenly you will start running 10K races each weekend or swim 1 mile each day in the pool. Unless you have been training all your life for a sport, it does not make sense to start something new at age 74. People who are sedentary all week, then attempt a heroic program on the weekends only are often referred to as "Weekend Warriors." We think this is not a good idea and could lead to medical problems. Certainly, you can, but why not start a program of organized, regular walking? This can be done seasonally outdoors in most parts of the country and transferred indoors to a treadmill as the weather dictates. Dr. Art Weltman, Chairperson of the Kinesiology Department at the University of Virginia has recommended fast-paced walking as the best and easiest form of exercise. He also found that women who do three short (30-minute) high-intensity walks, plus two moderately paced recovery walks a week, actually lose up to six times as much abdominal fat as a participant who simply strolls 5 days a week. Power walking is easier on the joints than running. When you walk, one foot is always in contact with the ground, while during jogging, there is a float stage in which the whole body in lifted in the air. When the person comes back down, the body is subjected to impact. For what it is worth, strolling (walking at a window-shopping pace) burns about 238 calories per hour, while brisk walking burns up to 340 calories per hour. Power walking, including using your arms to propel yourself forward, can burn more than 500 calories per hour. If you can, add hills (or increase the incline on a treadmill). There can never be an excuse for not walking. You can socialize with a friend or two and solve all the problems in the world. You can use wireless headphones to listen to music, sports, talk shows, or even financial news stations. Just do it!

2. *"I used to like swimming, but I now find it boring. Should I force myself to get into the pool?"*

Many people who have not been swimmers all their lives find it hard to develop and sustain a program of swimming laps. Even though swimming may be the best overall exercise, you need to have access to a heated swimming pool, preferably chemical-free, and find a time when you can schedule a lane. Certain seasons can cause the pool to become crowded. Swimming is considered a no-impact exercise, forces a person to extend the back, and can burn as many calories as one wants, depending upon how fast that person swims. However, swimming can be a lonely sport. You cannot talk to anyone while you swim, and wireless headphones are not always effective. The reason that people often quit swimming is boredom. Walking in a swimming pool against the resistance of the water is an option, especially if you can find a partner to walk with you.

3. ***"Should I join a gym? What should I look for before I sign up?"***
   According to a report in the AARP Bulletin (May 2022), the United States has more gyms (over 32,000) than it has McDonald's, Dunkin' Donuts, and Taco Bells combined. Research from the lab of Dr. Chris Sciamanna (Ludwig *et al.*, 2021) at the Penn State College of Medicine indicated that people who lived fewer than 3.7 miles from their gyms went five times or more per month. Those who drove more than 5 miles went just once. Joining a gym that one of your friends uses is also a good idea. Having a fitness partner can be motivating. Realize that most gym-goers are between 18 and 54, so expect that gyms to be most crowded before and right after work. Most gyms offer classes, equipment, or studios that you may never use. These include indoor pools, spinning classes, saunas, drink bars, and other high-tech machines. Maybe you do not need to pay for those services if you never plan to use them.

4. ***"What would be the best events in the gym? Should I hire a personal trainer? What should I expect to spend?"***
   Gyms usually contain a whole set of fitness machines such as treadmills, stair-climbing machines, elliptical machines, recumbent stationary bikes, erect stationary bikes, and bikes with video screens to simulate an outdoor riding experience. Rowing machines and various types of spinning bikes might be available. All of these are effective. Gyms also have resistance areas to work on bodybuilding machines, free weights, and stretching devices. If a person has not been a frequent gym attendee, much less a "gym rat," getting started is often a challenge. Do not try to do things without supervision. It is far better to hire a trainer in this situation. A person might start with 2 days a week for 3 to 4 months to get going. A trainer will certainly show a person how to use the machines or weights and should push an individual farther than the person would do things on her or his own, but the real value of a trainer is to be a "motivator," providing you with the encouragement to "show up." Just be careful that you find a trainer who is used to working with a person

your age. You don't want to get hurt while working out. Leaving the gym after a hard workout is a great feeling. The hourly rate for trainers varies from gym to gym, but you can expect to spend between $50 and $150 per hour, depending on the gym.

5. **"Is it a good idea to exercise with someone like a spouse, partner, or close friend?"**

Yes, for sure. First, you will not have an excuse not to show up on the street, in the car, or on the bike. You do not want to stand-up a friend. Second, you will probably do more with a friend (spouse or partner) than you might do yourself. Obviously, if you are an established walker, and someone new who joins you is a beginner, you will probably have a less intense workout, but talking to someone seems to make time pass more quickly.

6. **"How can I judge if I am pushing myself in aerobic exercise? Is using a heart rate monitor while exercising a good idea?"**

As discussed earlier in this chapter, you should train at 60–80% of your maximal heart rate. That number is a good rule of thumb. You can take your heart rate manually by lightly touching the area of your wrist just before your hand. You should be able to feel your pulse there. Count for 15 seconds and multiply by 4, and you will get your heart rate. Some machines have built-in heart rate monitors that get activated when your hands are in a certain place on that machine. You can use a watch, like an Apple watch or a Samsung watch, and both have heart rate options. You can buy a fitness watch, like the ones made by Garmin or FitBit. All these devices are affordable and have many more features than you will ever use. Just make sure that if you buy one in an electronics store that someone should show you how to use it. Some are even water-proof. These watches become "addicting" when you are trying to stay in shape. Some of the watches even have a program that will keep track of the total number of steps you walk each day and signal to you when you have reached 10,000 steps or whatever you set as your target goal.

7. **"I would like to exercise outdoors, but it is often too cold or too hot where I live. What can I do in my home? Should I have home exercise equipment installed?"**

If you have room in your house or apartment for an indoor piece of equipment and can afford the purchase price, then buying your own is definitely an option. Make sure you use it, however. Having something at home is certainly more convenient, but using the same device every day can be very boring. Many people buy equipment for home use that eventually becomes places to hang clothes before they reach the closet. If you do buy something, make sure that someone comes to your house to install the machine as some are harder to assemble than others.

8. ***"Is it a good idea to switch events from time to time, such as from cycling to elliptical machines, or swimming to treadmill?"***
   We are not sure that there are any studies that can answer that question. It seems reasonable to switch off from time to time, if, for no other reason than you will work out different muscle groups. An example of that might be outdoor bike riding on Monday, Wednesday, and a longer ride on Sunday. Then try a workout on the elliptical machine on Tuesday, Thursday, and Saturday, and swim laps on Friday. Just try to find a combination that works for you.

9. ***"Do you have any suggestions to help me 'just get out and do it'?"***
   Self-motivation is always the best, but sometimes motivation occurs only after a scare. Suffering a near heart attack or finding out from your doctor that your blood sugar level is too high, and you remember that your father had the same thing and died when he was 62. Another motivation might be the way you look in an outfit you bought less than a year ago, or your last child is getting married in 6 months, and you want to look good in the pictures. This is why it is best to find a friend, a spouse, or a partner who will exercise together with you. Fear works, as does a friend.
   An anecdote to share: Many, many years ago, the husband of one of my patients entered a contest with six friends. They were all males in their 50s, and each was more than 50 pounds overweight. They each put in $10,000, and the winner-take-all was the one who lost the greatest percentage of weight after 6 months. They all chose their own diet and exercise program. My patient's husband actually won the wager and pocketed $60,000. Of course, as soon as the competition was over, the contestants each resumed their "normal" eating and exercising pattern. As you probably have guessed by now, within the next 6 months they were each back to their pre-morbid weight. Within 4 years my patient's husband had died of a heart attack. Whatever program you chose, it should be one that you can stay on for the rest of your life.

10. *"If I have not exercised before, should I start out with an intense program?"*

   If you are a Baby Boomer and have not exercised regularly most of your life, especially if you know you have a cardiac condition, hypertension, and/or diabetes, you should first see your health care provider for a full evaluation. You might need to have a stress test to see how your body tolerates exercise. Your provider might also suggest a Calcium heart score to see if you have calcifications in the blood vessels of your heart. If you pass your tests, start slowly, and work up. Walking in your neighborhood, especially with a partner, works fine, as does walking on a treadmill. Walking in a swimming pool can also be advantageous. If you can afford a personal trainer, that person can work with you. Also, many hospitals have cardiac rehabilitation programs in which a therapist works specifically with people who have known heart disease. Just do it!

11. *"Do you have any theories as to why intense exercise may promote longevity?"*

   A speculation might be that intense exercise is associated with an increase in heart rate and more blood pushed around the circulation. More blood means more oxygen being carried to all the tissues in the body, including the brain. One, relatively uncommon, form of dementia is called "vascular dementia," and is associated with atherosclerosis in the brain. Vascular dementia differs from that associated with Alzheimer's disease in that patients who suffer from vascular dementia tend to involve speed of thinking and problem-solving rather than memory loss. Similar to atherosclerosis of the heart, there is insufficient oxygen being carried to brain cells. Having more blood circulating to the brain just might be an explanation for reducing dementia.

12. *"What are the takeaway points about exercise?"*

   1. Exercise seems to be an important factor in promoting longevity.
   2. The more intensely you exercise, the better off you are.
   3. Concentrate on cardio exercises, but don't forget weight training, flexibility, and balance work.
   4. Strongly consider having a personal trainer to help you get started and keep you going.

5. Exercise works for people with heart disease.
   Exercise works for people with diabetes.
   Exercise works for people with hypertension.
   Exercise works for people with early dementia.
   Exercise works for people with early Parkinson's disease.
   Exercise should work for everyone.
6. Strongly consider hiring a trainer to help you get started and keep motivated.
7. There are no excuses for not starting a program right now. It is never too late.

CHAPTER 3

Use Your Brain

One of the most crucial factors to facilitate longevity is continuing to use your brain.

For this chapter, we have broken the options down to two factors and have tried to present scientific studies to support our suggestions.

- Should you keep working as long as possible?
- If you do retire, should you take on a new career, even a voluntary one, to keep your brain active?

Does working longer help you live longer, or does it contribute to illness?

In the 1960s, 1970s and 1980s, men retired at age 65. "Full Retirement" as defined by the Social Security office was as follows:

Social Security Benefit Birth Year

Birth Year	Full Retirement Age
1943–1954	66
1955	66 years, 2 months
1956	66 years, 4 months
1957	66 years, 6 months
1958	66 years, 8 months
1959	66 years, 10 months
1960 and later	67 years

This meant that an individual could start receiving social security benefits at that age. Our fathers looked forward to that time in their lives where they could collect income from the government, not have to work, and have enough money to live on.

Starting around the 1990s or so, men began working longer than the recommended age of 65 to retire. The percentage of women in the workforce has dramatically changed since then, now to approximate that of men, and these women are also working longer.

Life expectancy for 65-year-old men in 1970 was 78 years; for 65-year-old women it was 82. Today, men and women who have reached the 65th birthday have life expectancies of 84 and 86, respectfully. If a person expects to live into his or her 80s, continuing to work as long as possible seems reasonable, especially if one does not have a viable plan for what to do with one's life if working is stopped.

In addition, multiple factors have changed working conditions. Factories now have robots. Retail shopping is slowly being replaced by online shopping. Office workers are often allowed to work from home. Manual labor is sometimes replaced by machinery. Even farming has become more mechanized. Professionals like lawyers and doctors have support from word processors and voice recognition technology. Call center jobs have replaced appointment staff. In short, jobs nowadays require less physical work, which means that many people have less physically demanding jobs, making it easier for them to continue working.

Add to that the cost of living, which has rapidly increased with inflation settling in. Many Baby Boomers, like us, do not have enough savings in their 401ks or retirement plans; nor do they have enough income from discretionary savings to use during retirement. This is another reason why some workers continue to work.

The last reason why so many are remaining at their jobs is that they are in better health than people of comparable age were a generation ago. Our fathers (most of us had stay-at-home mothers) looked forward to retirement at age 65 because they often had health problems to deal with and just got tired of working hard at their jobs. In addition, Baby Boomers quite often had more education, both college and postgraduate, than did their parents, and well-educated people tend to work longer in their chosen careers. Jobs once filled primarily by men are now filled equally by women (doctors, lawyers, accountants, pilots, etc.).

The U.S. Bureau of Labor Statistics reported in 2017 that 32% of people aged 65 to 69 were working, and 19% of people aged 70 to 74 were also employed. In 2021, 36% of people aged 65 to 69 continued to work, far more than the 22% who were working in 1994.

Even with those statistics about retirement age, many people still plan to "retire early." This trend toward early retirement along with several other ongoing demographic trends, including declining fertility rates, prolonged life expectancy, and delayed workforce entry by young adults, has contributed to a shrinking working population that may not be able to fiscally support a rapidly growing retired population. Leibfritz (2002) reported that to alleviate fiscal pressure on U.S. Social Security, the age eligibility for claiming full retirement benefits has been proposed to be increased from 65 to 67 years and benefits available at age 62 would be reduced. Most recently, research has pointed to a trend toward increased retirement age. Therefore, it is timely and critical to develop a better understanding of whether and how retirement age impacts retirees' health and longevity. Understanding the association of retirement age with longevity has important implications for postretirement survival and may elucidate criteria for evaluating the current policies that aim to encourage older workers to retire later and to remain in the workforce.

Wu *et al.* (2016) tried to understand the association of retirement age with longevity which has important implications for postretirement survival and may elucidate criteria for evaluating the current policies that aim to encourage older workers to retire later and to remain in the workforce. In their paper, over the study period of 18 years and 2,956 subjects, 234 healthy and 262 unhealthy retirees died, respectively. Among healthy retirees, a 1-year older age at retirement was associated with an 11% lower risk of all-cause mortality (95%), independent of a wide range of sociodemographic, lifestyle, and health confounders. Similarly, unhealthy retirees ($n = 1,022$) had a lower all-cause mortality risk when retiring later (Hazard ratio: 0.91, 95%). None of the sociodemographic factors were found to modify the association of retirement age with all-cause mortality. Their conclusion was that early retirement may be a risk factor for mortality while prolonged working life may provide survival benefits among U.S. adults.

Kachan *et al.* (2015) looked at National Health Interview Survey data from 1997 through 2011 for adults aged 65 or older ($n = 83,338$; mean age = 74.6 years). They tried to estimate the association of socioeconomic factors and health behaviors with four health status measures:

1. Self-rated health (fair/poor vs. good/very good/excellent)
2. Multimorbidity (≤1 vs. ≥2 chronic conditions)
3. Multiple functional limitations (≤1 vs. ≥2)
4. Health and Activities Limitation Index (HALex) (below vs. above 20th percentile).

They observed that employees over age 65 were projected to make up approximately 22% of the U.S. workforce by 2022. This population group is becoming increasingly diverse, with a growing proportion of racial/ethnic minorities and women, and the increased rates of workforce engagement in this population can be associated with various health outcomes. Older workers are a valuable addition to the workplace because they are on average just as productive as their younger counterparts; in addition, older workers are more careful and emotionally stable and demonstrate lower rates of absenteeism at work than their younger counterparts. There was, however, a lack of nationally representative studies comparing the effects of various sociodemographic, health behavior, and occupational factors on the health status of older workers and nonworkers.

They concluded that, compared to people who retired at or before age 65, people who continued to work past that age, were about three times more likely to report being in good health and about half as likely to have serious health problems, such as heart disease or cancer.

Goforth (2021) stated that other studies have linked working past retirement age with a reduced risk of dementia and heart attacks. However, there is quite a bit of variability in those observations.

Some people may have extreme stress on a job, which is a risk factor for coronary artery disease. Think of a physician, an attorney, a police officer, a money manager, an air traffic controller, or an airplane pilot, all of them have very stressful jobs.

Some jobs are extremely physically challenging. Think of a professional athlete, especially in a high-contact sport, or a coal miner, a stonemason, an iron or steel worker, a construction worker, a hard laborer, or a professional dancer. These jobs, in some cases, are so demanding that people can only last 5 to 10 years at them.

If an employee lacks meaning from his or her work, is constantly bored, or feels "burned out," all these may add stress to the employee's life.

Westerlund et al. (2010) studied over 14,000 people and found a different conclusion, looking at self-reported respiratory disease, type 2 diabetes, coronary artery disease, and stroke. They looked at patients seven years before and seven years after retirement and found no changes in the intensity or frequency of those chronic diseases. However, they did find a major reduction in mental and physical fatigue and depressive symptoms, particularly among people with chronic disease after retirement.

The conclusion of all these studies is that so much depends upon the individual person, but the tendency is that continuing to work longer, if you do not have serious medical conditions, is consistent with increased longevity.

What should you do? Be smart about your job. Don't remain at a job you hate, that you resent going to every day, or where your boss does not appreciate you. But, if you like what you do, if you feel you are making a difference in the lives of other people, or if you are earning a nice salary, then work as long as you can. A happy employee will live longer.

If you do retire, do not drop out of life. If you feel you want to travel, to explore new places, take up new hobbies, or become more involved in the lives of your children or grandchildren, do it. Don't lie around and do nothing! That gets stale quickly. Find something that you like to do, that you are good at, and that gives you the opportunity to help other people. You will be very happy with that choice. If you must work to earn money to live on during retirement, do that as well. If you want to volunteer, there are plenty of opportunities to do so, especially if you were good at certain things and can continue to use your skills. Volunteer at organizations you believe in. Take on responsible positions. Learn a new career or trade. Maybe even start a new company, not necessarily for making more money, but for the challenge, as well as the sense of accomplishment and satisfaction that can keep you motivated. Working at something you enjoy often does not seem like work.

If working at your job seems to contribute to longevity, does keeping your mind active and trying to learn new things have any effect on staying healthy or living longer?

Chen *et al.* (2010), neurobiologists at University of California, Irvine, reported that learning promotes brain health and, therefore, mental stimulation could limit the debilitating effects of aging on memory and the mind. They suggested that everyday forms of learning animate neuron receptors that help keep brain cells functioning at optimum levels. These receptors are activated by a protein called *brain-derived neurotrophic factor* (BDNF), which facilitates the growth and differentiation of the connections, or synapses, responsible for communication among neurons. BDNF is key in the formation of memories. They suggest that staying mentally active as we age can keep neuronal BDNF signaling at a constant rate, which may limit memory and cognitive decline.

Krell-Roesch *et al.* (2017) wrote that engaging in mentally stimulating activities even in late life may decrease the risk of mild cognitive impairment. They looked at five specific types of mentally stimulating activities in late life: reading books, playing games, craft activities, computer use, and social activities (going out to movies and theaters). These activities were associated with positive impact, although computer use seemed to have a larger effect than the others. They speculated that computer use may require specific technical and manual skills and that these could be factors that might be associated with a decreased risk of cognitive decline.

Zullo et al. (2019) reported that the mechanisms that extend life span in humans are poorly understood. They were able to show that extended longevity in humans is associated with a distinct transcription signature in the cerebral cortex that is characterized by downregulation of genes related to neural excitation and synaptic function. The transcription factor called "REST" is upregulated in humans with extended longevity and represses excitation-related genes. Transcription facts are proteins that switch genes on and off; that is, they control gene expression. Notably, REST-deficient mice exhibit increased cortical activity and neuronal excitability during aging. These findings reveal a conserved mechanism of aging that is mediated by neural circuit activity and regulated by REST. They concluded that altering neural activity can influence life span, as well as protecting the brain from stressful effects that damage nerve cells, such as those that lead to dementia.

Takeaway points:

1. Work as long as you desire, making retirement a personal choice, not a job mandate.
2. If you do retire, find something productive to do with your life: volunteer, change careers, start a new business, help your family, write a book, run a marathon, take up a new hobby, visit all seven continents. Do not sit around the pool at your condo and talk about all your friends or people on your condo board.
3. Keep involved with activities that stimulate your brain: reading, playing games, doing crafts, using your computer (don't be afraid to learn something new), and engaging in social activities.

There is enough scientific research to support all these suggestions.

CHAPTER 4

Socialization

The COVID-19 pandemic of 2019 to 2021 caused many problems for people around the world. Fear, illness, and death predominated our lives. While we waited for the virus to "burn itself out," or waited for the scientists to develop and distribute a vaccine to prevent us from becoming ill or dying, many of us realized that the virus was transmitted only by person-to-person contact, so the only way to remain safe was to stay away from other people. In addition, many cities and states had no choice but to force lockdowns. Schools, stores, restaurants, and offices closed, some voluntarily but most because of governmental orders. Only essential services were allowed to stay open, and most of us stayed in as much as possible. Even going out was a challenge, as we were almost afraid to come near another person for fear that person had COVID and could transmit it to us. It was during those times that many people began experiencing symptoms of social isolation and loneliness, especially those of us who live alone. We began to realize the importance of being with our family and friends. During the pandemic, about 4 in 10 adults in the U.S. reported symptoms of anxiety or depression, compared to 1 in 10 adults who reported those same symptoms between January and June 2019, as reported by the Kaiser Family Foundation (Panchal, *et al.*, 2021).

Experiences such as depression, anxiety, and suicidal thoughts were more prevalent during the COVID-19 pandemic, particularly for youth and young adults, caregivers, frontline workers, and Black, Indigenous, and People of Color (BIPOC) populations.

The question arose to us, "Does loneliness and social isolation affect longevity?"

In his book, *The Blue Zones: Lessons for Living Longer from the People Who've Lived the Longest*, Dan Buettner identified communities around the world where people live long, healthy lives. He observed that all these communities seemed to have a group of lifestyles that were present, to a great extent, in all the communities. Among those lessons, as he labeled them, were "Right Tribe" and "Community." The Right Tribe was a group of friends who committed to each other for life. They were always there for each other. The other important "lesson" he called "Community" in which the residents were all part of a community that offered social support and faith-based support during times of need. This study was clearly an observational one but did reveal especially important information.

Even before the COVID pandemic, it was known that risk factors for early mortality include a sedentary lifestyle, smoking, and air pollution. However, few studies ever explored social factors as a contributor to mortality. In a meta-analysis study, Holt-Lunstad *et al.* (2015) (Brigham Young University) attempted to explore the possibility that social factors might have an influence on emotional and physical well-being while contributing to a long life span. They looked at published studies that provided quantitative data on mortality as affected by loneliness, social isolation, or living alone. They looked at living alone, having few social network ties, and having infrequent social contact, all of which are markers of social isolation. Loneliness is the perception of social isolation or the subjective experience of being lonely. Another description of loneliness is the discrepancy between desired and actual social relationships. The results of this extensive study indicated that individuals lacking social connections are at risk of premature mortality. This averaged about 30% increased likelihood of mortality. The risk associated with social isolation and loneliness is comparable with well-established risk factors for mortality, including those identified with the U.S. Department of Health and Human Services (physical activity, obesity, substance abuse, responsible sexual behavior, mental health, injury and violence, environmental quality, immunization, and access to health care—https://www.hhs.gov/sites/default/files/surgeon-general-social-connection-advisory.pdf). A substantial body of research evidence has elucidated the psychological, behavioral, and biological pathways by which social isolation and loneliness lead to poorer health and decreased longevity. The authors felt that loneliness and social isolation lead to health issues similar to those that research on obesity observed over 30 years ago—that obesity is a major risk to health and well-being. They also concluded that affluent nations have the highest rates of individuals living alone, especially for adults over 65 years of age.

What suggestions can we offer to help people who suffer from loneliness and social isolation?

Dr. Stephanie Cacioppo, a psychologist and neuroscientist at the University of Chicago, says that loneliness is not about being physically surrounded by people. It is said that New York City is the loneliest place in the country, because one might feel especially lonely in a crowd. It is more about your mentality. When you feel lonely, it is usually because you are not satisfied with what you have, whether it is that moment, or throughout your life. Until you can identify and address what is your dissatisfaction, you will continue to feel isolated, left out, and in need of companionship.

Dr. Emma Seppala (2020) reported that loneliness is the leading reason people seek out therapy, and studies have indicated that loneliness in a risk factor for mortality. A brain imaging study showed that feeling ostracized activates our neural pain matrix. She recommends the following exercises for embracing loneliness:

Give the emotion full expression.
> Let the emotion take center stage. If you feel the emotion, it may just move through you more quickly.

Go into silence.
> Silence can be difficult and even scary for some people, but practice that with a time limit for that activity, in which you go for a walk alone or even a casual swim.

Engage in mindful meditation.
> Be with the sensations, thoughts, and emotions that arise without try-ing to control or change them. Start with a short meditation and work up to longer time.

Take care of your body.
> We often eat the wrong foods, consume too much alcohol, stay up too late, and forget to exercise. Do not assume that the body's well-being is independent of our mind. One of the best ways to take care of our minds is to take good care of our bodies.

Serve.
> Be kind, for everyone you meet is fighting a hard battle. There is always someone suffering more than you are. As Mother Teresa once said, "Help one person at a time, and always start with the person near-est you." Research has shown that compassion and service can be of tremendous benefit. Helping others can immediately change our per-spective and reenergize us. Mahatma Gandhi once wrote, "The best way to find yourself is to lose yourself in the service of others."

Here are some takeaways for you:

1. Cherish your spouse/partner. No matter how long you have been to-gether and how many disagreements you have had over the years,

you have each other to serve as a major support as you age. Never take each other for granted. Have a date night periodically where you each dress up and go out to someplace special together. Keep the sparks going! Just consider the consequences of not having each other.

2. Immediately following the loss of a spouse, the surviving spouse begins to feel loneliness, even if that person had months or years to prepare for the loss. This is sometimes called the "Broken Heart Syndrome." Nights and holidays seem to be the worst times. People soon cannot watch TV, read books, or go out alone. It becomes overwhelming to some. Anecdotally, and without scientific support, it is often seen that within one year after the first spouse passes away, especially if that person is over 85, the surviving spouse dies. Perhaps being alone is too strong a factor for that person to keep going.

3. Keep looking for a new partner if you are alone. At our ages, we don't remarry for children or to grow our assets. Relationships are often important for just companionship. It is tough to eat lunch and dinner alone every day (see how important food is in our lives). There are so many places to meet people nowadays—grocery stores, the gym, art museums, the train or airplane, and even the myriad of online dating sites for people our age. (Ask your kids to help sign you up.) Ask friends to introduce you to people who might share common interests and values with you. Don't be shy. Most likely, the person you meet might also be suffering from similar loneliness.

4. Keep working, maybe harder than ever. If you are still working at your job or career, keep at it, as long as possible. There is no good reason to retire, except if your company has a policy in writing of mandatory retirement at a certain age. Work is good for your brain, especially if you are good at what you do.

5. If work is behind you, consider volunteering. So many places would be happy to have you. Maybe you like children and volunteering at a daycare, preschool, elementary school, or high school might challenge you. Work as a volunteer in a hospital. Volunteer at your religious center, like your church, synagogue, or mosque. Volunteer at a museum, the local Boys and Girls Club, YMCA, JCC, or even get a job as a greeter at your local Walmart store. Find something to do with your time that you enjoy doing, something that you are good at, and something that allows you to help others. Even do a Google search for "Where can I volunteer in [name of your city or town]?"

6. Travel regularly if you can afford it. Cruises and organized trips are a great way to spend your time (and your money). All of those organized trips are used to having guests traveling alone. Even if you have to pay a premium for a single room, cruises are a great way to meet new people, as well as have a fabulous time and see places you have never visited or places you want to see again.

7. If you have moved out of the house where you reared your children and, perhaps, now live in an apartment or a condominium, take advantage of any activities available. There are places around the country that have relatively affordable housing for seniors like us and are known for their activities. They include theaters, concerts, lectures, movies, and even dancing. Most condo buildings have their own activities, so try to go to everything. Maybe even run for the board of your condo if you enjoy those things.

8. Be somewhat aggressive in saying hello to people in your gym or walking in your neighborhood or in a grocery store where you shop. Start saying nice things to people on the phone when you call your phone carrier because of an issue with your cellphone. Give compliments to the person who helps you on the phone when you are trying to book airline tickets and cannot figure out how to do it online, even if you had to wait over 1 hour on hold. Acknowledge the cashier at the grocery store where you shop or the person who waits on you at Starbucks. Being nice is contagious.

9. Last, consider asking your kids for advice. Maybe you could volunteer at their company or offer to help with your grandchildren if that is a geographic possibility. Make it clear to your children that meeting someone will not jeopardize what you will leave them in your will, something that is often a major issue in some families. Most children do want to see their parent happy.

In the future, we may have a solution for loneliness, especially for people who live in extended care facilities, like nursing homes. Often people who live there are bored with not much to do all day, especially those with mild-to-moderate dementia. At the Aspen Idea Health program in 2022, Professor Arshia Khan from the University of Minnesota-Duluth presented her work using robots to help nursing home patients with loneliness. Using artificial intelligence, the robot can actually communicate with a patient, ask and answer questions, and be a source of comfort for a lonely elderly person. Of course, much work in this area still needs to be done, like making the robot look more humanoid, sound more like a human, and incorporate touch, perhaps, but this work may prove valuable in the next ten years as the robotic technology improves.

Realize that the only way you can combat loneliness is to face it and do something about it. Make it a point to work on that every day.

CHAPTER 5

Spiritual Life

Is longevity affected by Spirituality or Stress? To answer that question, we turned to psychologists, then the Bible, and then to clergy for suggestions. In addition, we will make some comments about three practices that have been discussed as having the ability to prolong life: prayer, yoga, and meditation.

Andy Roman, M.S., LMHC, RN is a clinical psychologist and therapist who has worked at Hippocrates Wellness Center for over 30 years. We will start with his comments.

The Danish Twin Study (Herskind *et al.*, 1996) challenged the myth that longevity was dictated by our genes. The authors demonstrated that only about 20% comes from inheritance, whereas the other 80% is determined by our lifestyles and our environment. Lifestyle includes physical, mental, emotional, spiritual, and sociological practices. Our environment includes everything we eat or breathe, whom we socialize with, where we travel, and where we live. We must ask the questions, "How can we measure those factors? What shortens our life span? What can we do to lengthen it?"

Science has discovered many markers that are intended to measure how what we do affects our life span. One of those is telomere length. Telomeres are the chromatic structures at the tips of chromosomes (like the plastic tips of shoelaces) that maintain genome stability by preventing chromosome degradation. Telomere length correlates with longevity: The longer the telomeres, the longer the life. We can measure to a large degree what lengthens and what shortens our telomeres, and that applies to both mental and physical health practices.

Psychotherapists are fascinated with the role of the heart and the mind in the total health picture. Most studies report reduced telomere length in patients suffering from mental disorders compared to the general population. Vakonaki *et al.* (2018) showed that telomeres are significantly shorter in people with mood disorders, especially depression. Simon *et al.* (2006) found that life span-shortening not only applies to those diagnosed with mood disorders. Increased psychological and chronic stress, as commonly observed in modern society, but also to those suffering obesity, systemic inflammation, increased cortisol levels, and oxidative degradation—now, all of these are associated with accelerated aging and telomere length-shortening. Espel *et al.* (2009) reported that stress comes out in diverse ways and that mental health does a body good. The late Arthur Janov, Ph.D., creator of *Primal Therapy* once said: "It is clear that stress and its hand-maiden, cortisol, the stress hormone, does shorten telomeres. Our beginning patients were high in cortisol until one year of therapy; then it reduced significantly. We assume that since cortisol and telomeres work in see-saw fashion: cortisol high, telomeres short; cortisol low, telomeres longer. I am convinced that since we lower cortisol we may also lengthen telomeres, or at least keep them from shortening. When telomeres get too short so do our lives." He also felt that deep feeling integrative therapy lengthens our life span!

Telomere length, as measured in the immune cells (Lindqvist *et al.*, 2015), is the most telling of all. Shortened leukocyte telomere length (LTL) reflects a cell's history with cumulative inflammation and oxidation and correlates with shorter life span. It is in our blood; it affects us for a lifetime, and we can measure it. Now we know we can change it.

Numerous studies concur that telomeres shorten by:

- eating a poor-quality diet
- eating more calories than needed
- low vitamin D
- excessive internal and external stress (there's the mental health part of it!)
- pretty much anything else that we know isn't so healthy.

Bongiorno (2012) in his book, *How Come They're Happy and I'm Not? The Complete Natural Program for Healing Depression for Good*, discusses that unhealthy practices shorten telomeres. He, like many others, felt that unhealthy practices shorten telomeres. Even science is screaming for us to stop abusing our bodies, to cultivate healthy habits, and to connect with our inner life and mental health. It is time to listen to what science affirms and what our hearts know to be true.

Now let's look at who's getting it right: In his book, *The Blue Zone Dwellers: Lessons for Living Longer from the People Who've Lived the Longest* (2008), Dan Buettener described noteworthy subcultures or communities where not only is the average life span significantly longer than in other parts of the world but also where more individuals live into old age than other places. Let's see what four of the communities are doing right:

Okinawa, Japan

Okinawa boasts the highest number of centenarians per capita in the world! Gardening, as a widespread and common activity, brings older citizens the benefits of sunshine, exercise, and nutritious plant-based foods. Okinawans adhere to a philosophy that promotes eating in moderation, and never gorging. They consume a lot of seaweed. They also have a sense of purpose, a positive outlook on life, and close social support groups called "moais."

Nicoya Peninsula, Costa Rica

The prevalent mindset in this population encourages a lifestyle that is physically active, with plenty of time in nature as well as time spent on family and spirituality. They sleep 8 hours, and their diet includes not only nutrient-rich local fruits, beans, rice, and corn but also water that's naturally high in calcium and magnesium.

Ikaria, Greece

Home to mineral hot springs, Ikaria has been a health destination for decades. Its residents stay active through walking, farming, and boating, but they also take time out to nap and socialize. They supplement their Mediterranean diet with wild greens and drink a local nutrient-rich herbal tea. The community encourages good health habits and promotes regular social engagement.

Loma Linda, California, USA

Loma Linda, about 60 miles east of Los Angeles, CA, is a community of 23,000 that includes about 9,000 Seventh Day Adventists—a group that is significantly longer-lived than the average American. Adventist culture focuses on healthful habits such as vegetarianism and excludes alcohol, caffeine, and smoking. Adventists drink plenty of water, exercise regularly, and tend to maintain a healthy weight. They nurture emotional and spiritual health, value their family relationships, and prize volunteering.

Buettner found some common ingredients of these specific communities:

1. Right tribe
   The world's longest-lived people live in social and cultural circles that support healthy lifestyle habits, like diet and exercise.

2. Strong social networks

   This includes strong family ties. This means keeping aging parents and grandparents nearby or in the home (it lowers disease and mortality rates of children in the home too.). They commit to a life partner (which can add up to 3 years of life expectancy) and invest in their children with time and love.

3. Natural moving

   Lots of gardening! More generally: moving naturally, and a lot. No gym memberships or aerobic classes, but movement as a way of life.

4. Belonging

   A cooperative community spirit, often centered around a faith or a church.

5. Plant slant, moderation in eating, and no junk

   Primarily plant-based diets! A limited or zero consumption of refined sugar and other processed foods. The 80% Rule. Hara hachi bu— the Okinawan 2,500-year old Confucian mantra—said before meals reminds them to stop eating when their stomachs are 80% full. The 20% gap between not being hungry and feeling full could be the difference between maintaining healthy weight and being off mark. People in the Blue Zones eat their smallest meal in the late afternoon or early evening, and then, they do not eat any more the rest of the day

6. Seniors are valued as members of family and the community

   To be appreciated in older age helps a person live longer!

7. Downshifting

   Even people in the Blue Zones experience stress. Stress leads to chronic inflammation, associated with every major age-related disease. (The American Medical Association has noted that stress is the basic cause of more than 60% of all human illness and disease.) What the world's longest-lived people have that others do not are routines to shed that stress, such as prayer, taking naps, and happy hours.

8. Purpose.

   The Okinawans call it "Ikigai," and the Nicoyans call it "plan de vida." For both, it translates to "why I wake up in the morning." Knowing your sense of purpose is worth up to 7 years of extra life expectancy. Some studies also mention that Blue Zone dwellers (all but the Adventists) regularly partake in moderate alcohol consumption. Is that a contributing factor to longevity, or just a coincidence? (The World Health Organization has ruled there is no amount of alcohol that is healthy. That's why I didn't include it in the numbered points.) OK, those are some community and lifestyle factors in longevity. What about the personal, inner life traits or habits of people who live a long life?

The Longevity Project: Surprising Discoveries for Health and Long Life from the Landmark Eight-Decade Study, by Friedman and Martin (2012, Hudson Street Press), provides some surprising findings:

1. The strongest predictor of long life was conscientiousness, which is another word for self-responsibility. Conscientious people are less likely to smoke, engage in risky behavior, and have accidents, and they are more likely to focus on the big picture and make good health choices moment to moment.
2. Avoiding stress alone doesn't add up to longevity, but being engaged with meaningful work does. A sense of purpose far outweighs the absence of hassles. In fact, service to others ranked high in Friedman and Martin's study—even greater than feeling loved by others.
3. Being part of something bigger than yourself: Selfish people die younger than people who belong to a group or to a movement. That can be a church or a religion, a healthy lifestyle, or the peace corp. People who volunteer for something live longer than those who don't, but it has to be selfless work. (The science shows that people who volunteer only for their own personal satisfaction don't live any longer than people who don't volunteer at all.)
4. Humming and singing. Yes, humming and singing. The healthiest people in the world seem to intuitively know the value of oxygen and regularly practice deep breathing in some form or other. Rigorous daily exercise is one way; humming or singing, another. The happiness factor might play into that.
5. And, finally, the authors found that people over 100 years old laugh a lot. In fact, easy to laugh and laughing often, are two of the traits high on the longevity list.

Rabbi Berel Light of Sydney, Australia, shared with us some information about the recommendations in the Bible for living a long life. The Bible was written by Moses at the direction of G-d around the year 1,450 BCE. Even back then people must have been interested in what might be done to prolong their lives. There are specifically two acts for which we are promised the reward, "that it should be good for you, and you should lengthen your days."

The first is found in the Ten Commandments. The fifth of the Ten Commandments says, "Honor your father and your mother, as the Lord your God commands you; so that your days will be long and it will be well for you" (Deuteronomy, 5:15). Although this specifically mentions one's parents, it also has been interpreted as honoring one's human parents is compared to honoring G-d.

The second act is a little more difficult to understand. It is found in Deuteronomy, 22:6. "If a bird's nest chances before you on the road, on any tree, or on the ground, and [it contains] fledglings or eggs, if the mother is sitting upon the fledglings or upon the eggs, you shall not take the mother [from] the upon the young. You shall send away the mother, and [then] you may take the young for yourself, in order that it should be good for you, and you should lengthen your days." This is a difficult passage to understand. It may be a Divine decree for which no reason is given. It may refer to teaching humans the trait of compassion since we are saving the mother bird from witnessing us taking her young. It may be that it teaches us about preservation of the species, since even though we are taking the offspring, the mother is still free to lay more eggs (Rambam). Regardless of the interpretation, the passage does mention living longer.

These two acts tell us that human beings are provided recommendations that might be able to extend their lives by living their spiritual lives in a certain way.

We now ask, can prayer make a difference? Going to church (or synagogue or mosque) is easier to measure than the intimate, individual way a person might practice religion (Ducharme, 2018). The research on praying has been mixed. Six studies have demonstrated a reduction in mortality for frequent church attenders, even after controlling for demographics, health, social, and psychological factors known to impact mortality (House et al., 1982; Hummer et al., 1999; Koenig et al., 1999; Oman & Reed, 1998; Strawbridge et al., 1997; Zuckerman et al., 1984). Another study (Helm et al., 2000) looked at a large number of elderly subjects. Their conclusion was that there was a significant protective effect against mortality for private religious activity in a relatively healthy elderly population, even after controlling for multiple confounding variables. They also suggested that increased prayer occurs in response to stress; however, those who waited until they developed declining health to begin prayer may be too late to show a protective effect against mortality.

A different study (Benson et al., 2006) found that people who knew they were being prayed for (intercessory prayer) before undergoing open heart surgery was associated with a higher incidence of complications.

Tyler J. VanderWeele, Ph.D., who is the John L. Loeb and Frances Lehman Loeb Professor of Epidemiology in the Departments of Epidemiology and Biostatistics at the Harvard T.H. Chan School of Public Health, and Director of the Human Flourishing Program and Co-Director of the Initiative on Health, Religion and Spirituality at Harvard University, was a coauthor of a paper (Shanshan *et al.*, 2016) looking at 74,534 women in the Nurses' Health Study who were free of cardiovascular disease and cancer at baseline. The authors' conclusions were robust in sensitivity and concluded that religion and spirituality may be an underappreciated resource that physicians could explore with their patients, as appropriate.

Another study (Bruce *et al.*, 2017) found a significant association between church attendance and mortality among middle-aged adults. They also found that regular service attendance was linked to reductions in the body's stress responses and even in mortality—so much so that worshippers were 55% less likely to die during the 18-year follow-up period than people who did not frequent the church, synagogue, or mosque.

In addition to the comments and suggestions made by a psychologist, a clergyperson, and research about prayer, we feel that there are two other areas of spirituality that needs to be explored: yoga and meditation.

Many Baby Boomers are constantly looking for ways to look and feel younger, in addition to ways to live longer. We drink smoothies and green drinks, use facial creams with or without hormones or other growth factors in them, and even consider cosmetic surgery, things that our parents did not even know about, much less considered using.

Yoga is a Hindu practice. Yoga comes from the root word "yuj" in Sanskrit, means to unite. Most Hindu texts discuss yoga as a practice to control the senses and the mind. The most famous is the Bhagavad Gita (dating back to 6th-3rd century BCE), in which Krishna speaks of four types of yoga—*bhakti*, or devotion; *jnana*, or knowledge; *karma*, or action; and *dhyana*, or concentration (often referred to as *raja yoga*, though not all sources agree on the term)—as paths to achieve *moksha*, the ultimate goal, according to Hindu understanding. Many Boomers, and even many people who are much younger, participate in yoga classes of all types. There are so many yoga studios appearing all over, and many people who practice this skill are extremely flexible in the movement of their bodies. If you have never visited or taken a class, when you do so, you will be amazed at how flexible some people are. Yoga might be something for some of you to consider. People constantly say that at the end of a class you might find a more relaxed state of mind, better sleep, or more energy.

Some people say that Western medicine is uncovering clues about this ancient practice.

What are the benefits of yoga? According to Mary Hazen (2015), they include the following:

1. Prevent cartilage and joint breakdown
2. Increases bone density and health
3. Increase blood
4. Cleanses lymph and immune systems
5. Ups your heart rate (in some classes, while slows your heart rate in others)
6. Regulates your adrenal glands (*i.e.,* lowers cortisol levels)
7. Lowers your blood sugar and bad cholesterol (LDL)
8. Improves your balance
9. Calms your nervous system and help you sleep deeper
10. Give your lungs room to breathe
11. Improves your digestion
12. Encourages self-care and healthy lifestyle

According to Wikipedia, Meditation is a practice in which an individual uses a technique—such as mindfulness, or focusing the mind on a particular object, thought, or activity—to train attention and awareness and achieve a mentally clear and emotionally calm and stable state.

Meditation is practiced in numerous religious traditions. The earliest records of meditation (dhyana) are found in the Upanishads, and meditation plays a salient role in the contemplative repertoire of Jainism, Buddhism, and Hinduism. Since the 19th century, Asian meditative techniques have spread to other cultures where they have also found application in nonspiritual contexts, such as business and health.

Meditation may significantly reduce stress, anxiety, depression, and pain and enhance peace, perception, self-concept, and well-being. Research is ongoing to better understand the effects of meditation on health (psychological, neurological, and cardiovascular) and other areas.

For many of us who have never attempted meditation before, we just think of meditation as the cross-legged pose with your arms resting on your lap and your hands forcing a circle by touching your index fingers to your thumbs. As in yoga, there are many types of meditation that people practice. Some mediators practice a specific type of meditation like Transcendental Meditation (TM) or Shamatha Meditation, but meditation can be as simple as starting your day with a few minutes of silence and mindfulness and may even be things like going on a long run alone, a long-distance bike ride (of course, using an e-bike), watching the waves rush in and out at a beach, skiing alone on fresh powder, looking at a crackling fire in a fireplace, walking through a silent rain forest, swimming laps in a swimming pool, or a long car drive through the mountains. You can even meditate using an app that can guide you through your journey. There is no "best" type of meditation, only the one that works the best for you.

Again, as with yoga, there are science-based benefits of meditation (Thorpe & Link, 2020):

1. Reduces stress
2. Controls anxiety
3. Promotes emotional health
4. Enhances self-awareness
5. Lengthens attention span
6. May reduce age-related memory loss
7. Can generate kindness
8. May help fight addictions
9. Improves sleep
10. Helps control pain
11. Can decrease blood pressure
12. Accessible anywhere

Now, we need to explore the science. Are there any published studies that address whether yoga or meditation can lengthen your life expectancy?

An early study (Alexander et al., 1990) looked at 73 residents living in 8 nursing homes who were randomly assigned, between no-treatment group and three experimental groups, to the following programs: transcendental meditation (TM) program, mindfulness training (MF), or relaxation. At the end of three years, the survival rate for the TM group was 100% and 87% for the MF group, with a much lower rate of survival for the other groups.

The next few studies looked at telomere length. As we discussed earlier in this chapter, telomere length is one of the possible biomarkers for longevity. Telomeres are nucleoprotein structures located at the ends of chromosomes which shorten with repetitive dell division and replication (Hoge et al., 2013). Telomeres shorten with age, and this shortening may be accelerated in the presence of cellular oxidative damage or chronic psycho-logical stress (Damjanovic *et al.*, 2007). Shorter telomeres have been linked to chronic stress. Specific lifestyle behaviors that can mitigate the effects of stress might be associated with longer telomere lengths. Previous research has suggested that there might be a link between behaviors that focus on the well-being of others—such as volunteering and caregiving—and overall health and longevity.

Hoge *et al.* (2013) looked at relative telomere length, as noted earlier in this chapter, in a group of individuals experienced in Loving-Kindness Medi-tation (LKM), a practice derived from the Buddhist tradition that utilizes a focus on unselfish kindness and warmth toward all people, using control par-ticipants who did no meditation. The researchers looked at relative telomere length in 15 LKM practitioners and 22 control participants. Their conclusion was that the LKM practitioners had significantly longer telomere length than controls. They suggested the intriguing possibility that LKM practice might alter telomere length.

Another study (Tolahunase *et al.*, 2017) looked at several biomarkers of cellular aging and metabotrophic biomarkers in subjects who were intro-duced to Yoga and Meditation–based lifestyle intervention (YMLI). They first acknowledged that there are currently no "gold standards" for these biomarkers, but used cellular DNA damage, telomere length attrition, and oxidative stress as biomarkers of cellular aging. They used other biomarkers of stress and inflammatory response, neuroplasticity, and longevity. After 12 weeks of YMLI, there were significant improvements in both the cardinal biomarkers of cellular aging and the metabotrophic biomarkers influencing cellular aging compared to baseline values.

Levine *et al.* (2017) published results in the *Journal of the American Heart Association*, suggesting that there is a possible benefit on cardiovascular risk, although the quantity of study data is modest.

As noted throughout this chapter, telomere shortening has been asso-ciated with age-related conditions and telomere length is hypothesized to be a biomarker of aging and age-related morbidity. DNA methylation changes have been described at specific subtelomeric regions in long-term meditators. Mendioroz *et al.* (2020) showed no association with telomere length in the group of long-term meditation. Their results may suggest that long-term meditation could be related to epigenetic mecha-nisms, in particular gene-specific DNA methylation changes at distinct regions.

All of these studies still are not totally conclusive because of certain factors. The study we need to definitely conclude that yoga and/or meditation will include the following:

Utilize a randomized study design
Blinded adjudication of endpoints
Adequate power to meet the primary study outcome(s)
Include long-term follow-up
Have <20% dropout rate
Have <85% follow-up data
Be performed by investigators without inherent financial or intellectual bias in outcome

The conclusion of this chapter is that spirituality seems very important. To have a belief in a higher power and to express it with regular religious services may be particularly important. To follow the suggestions of the Bible makes sense, as do practices of yoga and meditation

Keep Having Sex

Baby Boomers helped start the "sexual revolution" of the 1960s in the United States. During that time, social norms changed as sex became more widely discussed in society. Erotic media, such as films, magazines, and books, were appearing. The development of the oral contraceptive pill ("the pill") in 1960 might have initiated this revolution, as women gained more control of their bodies and sexuality. The women's liberation (women's lib) movement also appeared during that time, providing sexual freedom to women for the first time.

During that time sexual freedom and morals began to quickly change. There were communes with "free sex," there was abundant sex on college campuses, and premarital sex became the norm. There was the Woodstock concert in upstate New York. A common event was "free love," a liberal philosophy that sought freedom from state regulation and church interference in personal relationships. There was even a famous song promoting "Drugs, sex, rock and roll." Many Baby Boomers participated in that revolution, some more than others. Sex became a very important part of their lives.

What has happened 60 or so years later?

A survey from the American Association of Retired People (AARP) of 1,816 people showed:

71% say sex is still important to their lives.
54% are satisfied with their sex lives.
67% admit that their sexual desire has receded in the past 20 years.
45% of Baby Boomers are less comfortable with their appearance than 10 years before.

It appears that many Baby Boomers feel that sex was and still is an important part of their lives. However, some situations may have developed over the years that could affect their sexual abilities. Some have developed medical conditions as they have aged. Some consume too much alcohol, which can cause erection problems in men and delay orgasms in women.

Some have arthritis making the act of sex uncomfortable. We might have chronic pain, early dementia, depression, or diabetes, all of which contribute to sexual dysfunction. Some have cardiovascular disease and worry that sexual activity could precipitate a new cardiac event. Many take medications, some of which can cause erectile dysfunction, difficulty with ejaculation, difficulty with libido, and vaginal dryness. Some of these are medications used for treating high blood pressure, some are antihistamines, some are antidepressants, and some are ulcer meds. For sure, before trying to increase your sexual activity, please be evaluated by your primary doctor or cardiologist.

Yet, the Internet is full of claims of the benefits of regular sex. Some of those benefits include:

1. Helps keep the immune system humming
2. Boosts libido
3. Improves a women's bladder control
4. Lowers blood pressure
5. Counts as exercise
6. Lowers heart attack risk
7. May make prostate cancer less likely
8. Improves sleep
9. Eases stress
10. Maintains vaginal blood flow and vaginal health

A different review in WebMD said that the sex life of an average person used to be thought to end at age 70 (Warner, 2010). However, life experiences have shown that people tend to want and have sex till they have their last breath. Lindau and Gavrilova (2010) reported that people of sound health reported interest in sex regardless of their age group.

> 39% of men and 17% of women were sexually active in the 75-85-year-old age group. 71% of those who were sexually active had a good quality sex life.

Men and women who reported very good or excellent health were more likely to be sexually active compared with their peers who were in poor health. There are many factors to explain that observation, including the loss of a partner and other underlying medical conditions. The proportion of sexually active elderlies could considerably increase if seniors that have solo sex are considered, particularly as studies have suggested that masturbation is common in older adults. The authors also estimated the average remaining years of sexually active life gained as a result of good health using a new health expectancy indicator for clinical and public health application. Their research showed that men in good or excellent health participated in regular sexual activity lived an extra five to seven years, and women in substantially good health lived three to six years longer. Even though the gender gap is evident, the research provided a clear association between health and sexual activity. As we have said before, this study, like many others, is an observational one based on surveys, not a prospective one following patients for 20 to 30 years, something that may never be done.

Even if it seems logical that being in better health should contribute to longevity (which we feel it does), we are still trying to answer the question, is there any scientific evidence behind continuing to be sexually active can make a difference in longevity?

To help us answer that question, we have turned to an expert, Alan Altman, M.D., Assistant Clinical Professor of Obstetrics, Gynecology, and Reproductive Biology at Harvard Medical School and Past President of the International Society for the Study of Women's Sexual Health (ISSWSH), the largest multidisciplinary international professional society devoted solely to female sexual function and dysfunction.

Use it or lose it:
The health of a woman's sex organs depends on maintaining healthy blood flow to the vagina, the labia, and the clitoris. Blood flow brings oxygen and nutrients to these important structures and helps keep them functioning. Blood flow also helps maintain the elasticity of the vagina, both inside and out, and produces lubrication so that intercourse does not become painful when the vagina is stretched by penile penetration. Blood flow to the labia and clitoris is important for arousal and orgasm during which those structures become swollen and sensitive to stimulation. When any kind of sexual stimulation occurs, whether partnered or self-stimulated as with masturbation, the brain sends increased blood flow to all these structures. Thus, "use it or lose it" means that any sexual activity will increase blood flow to these vital structures, which, in turn, help maintains their health and functioning. Hence, any sexual activity can help keep a woman sexual longer and more successfully! A list of what can be included in "any sexual activity" might include vaginal intercourse, vaginal outercourse (especially if a male partner has a degree of erectile dysfunction and is unable to successfully penetrate), masturbation with or without

sex toys, watching sexually stimulating movies or videos, and even use of a "sexbot" (life-like sexual robots that are becoming more sophisticated and responsive at this writing). So, anything that will sexually arouse a woman will increase blood flow and help maintain sexual function.

Estrogen:
Even with increases in blood flow during stimulation and arousal, over time, especially many years after menopause, blood flow naturally diminishes, thereby reducing lubrication and vaginal elasticity. Less blood flow also makes orgasm longer to achieve and lowers the peak feeling of release and pleasure. That's where estrogen comes in. Appropriate postmenopausal use of estrogen has many benefits on heart, brain, bone, blood vessels, skin, mucous membranes, joints, the immune system, the vulva, vagina, and bladder (pretty important structures and organs!). Using systemic (throughout the body) or local estrogen (just affecting the vagina) can maintain the necessary blood flow indefinitely! The biggest cause of loss of sexual desire in women as they age is painful intercourse due to vaginal atrophy or loss of elasticity in the vagina secondary to diminished blood flow. And who wants to have sex if it hurts? So, the loss of sex drive. Estrogen can help avoid and even correct this vaginal atrophy when it occurs. It should be mentioned that vaginal lubricants available over the counter can also be quite helpful when dryness first begins to occur to diminish pain associated with early vaginal atrophy, but as time goes on, many will need estrogen to recapture the lost lubrication and elasticity.

Spontaneous desire versus responsive desire:
As women age, and especially the longer they are with the same partner, spontaneous desire (wanting to rip his or her clothes off and have sex on the kitchen table) can naturally diminish over time. Thankfully, this loss of *spontaneous desire* often transitions over to *responsive sexual desire*. This means that she will need to be stimulated and aroused before the desire sets in. Let me explain further. The phases of sexual response in men and women, as described by Masters and Johnson, traditionally start with desire (being "turned on") which then leads to arousal followed by orgasm. Over the past few decades, women's sexual response phases have been described differently than those of men. Instead of desire needing to precede arousal, sometimes arousal must occur before the desire sets in. In other words, her desire occurs in "response" to becoming aroused

instead of spontaneously before she is aroused, hence the term "responsive desire." Countless patients have come to my practice complaining of loss of sexual desire and wanting to "get it back." On questioning, they report that they'd just as soon read a good book than have sex! Many women will have sex with their partner just to keep the partner happy and the relationship close despite not having the desire to do so in the first place. But on further questioning, most of them admit that after they allow themselves to become aroused by their partner stimulating them, they then get turned on and want to continue to a "happy ending!" When I explain to them that they are taking the responsive desire route, and that this is a perfectly normal transition which does not indicate any problem, and that there will still be times when spontaneous desire may occur, they thank me and leave feeling quite normal and far more confident. It should also be mentioned that there is a new generation of medications that have been developed to enhance women's sex drive and recently approved for use by prescription under appropriate indications by physicians with experience in female sexual function and dysfunction (Addyi and Vyleesi).

Testosterone use:
The "male hormone" testosterone is also important in women, principally because all the natural estrogen called estradiol, made by the ovaries before menopause sets in, comes from testosterone made by the ovaries which is then turned into estradiol by enzymes present in those same ovaries! Testosterone is also responsible for bone health, muscle strength, mood, sex drive, and arousal. So many women will ask for testosterone because they believe that it will help keep their sex drive active and spontaneous, as they have heard it does in men. After menopause, the ovaries no longer make the natural estradiol, which is why menopause occurs, but they still produce testosterone for another decade or two, so testosterone may not be as necessary as estrogen is after menopause. Also, through many years of practice, I have found that estrogen replacement post-menopause will frequently increase sex drive without the need for additional testosterone. In the smaller percentage of women who might still need testosterone added to their hormonal regimen, it should be carefully prescribed considering the potential male-like problems, such as hair growth, scalp hair loss, voice changes, and clitoral enlargement that might occur with high doses of testosterone. More importantly, however, women who have had their ovaries surgically removed are missing

the testosterone that is still made by the ovaries as explained above after menopause and, therefore, are the best candidates for addition of testosterone to their hormone regimen to help maintain sexual function.

Does sex help longevity or does longevity help sex?

While the above suggestions can help maintain a woman's ability to continue to experience a longer and happier sex life, the question remains: Will a longer and happier sex life actually help her live longer? Many articles in the lay press have claimed that continuing to have sex into the "elder years" helps people live longer and healthier lives! There has even been a scientific paper published by scientists in California (of course!) showing that the protective caps on our DNA, which indicate aging and general health, are in better shape in women who have "weekly romps!" These caps, called telomeres, keep our DNA in shape and stop our chromosomes from fraying as we get older. Natural aging shortens the caps, and it is known in the medical literature that shorter telomeres mean a shorter life span. These researchers found significantly longer telomeres in women who said they had weekly sexual intimacy (de Baca *et al.*, 2017) So, the question remains, do women with more sex have longer telomeres, or do women with longer telomeres have more sex as they age? This is yet to be definitively determined!

A few more important points:

I am often asked about the "normal" frequency of sexual relations or masturbation in older people. The answer is that everyone has a different "normal!" Try not to measure yourself and your sex life by what others may claim. Measure yourself by what you have been used to in the past. The best indicator of whether sexual satisfaction will continue into the later years is how satisfying sex has been prior to those years.

Patients also want to know, "What's more important—the act of intercourse or the emotional feelings associated with the closeness or having an orgasm?" My answer is—all of these contribute to a happy and successful sex life, and the closeness engendered in sexual activity is the more important result in our human species. The act of vaginal penetrative intercourse is frequently not possible as we age and, hence, the importance of "outercourse" where there is sex play without penetration. Also, as orgasm becomes less achievable, satisfaction often takes its place due to the closeness that remains achievable.

Finally, losing one's spouse/partner is an unfortunate reality as we age and has an obvious and direct impact on sexual intimacy and activity.

I have had several patients describe feeling guilt about continuing their sexual lives either through masturbation or seeking another partner. Others have said that it's simply a time to stop. This situation is becoming more common as we live longer into the 90s and even beyond. The level of sexual closeness achieved in a couple's lifetime is often related to the seeking out of another partner to help recapture the missed closeness experienced prior to the loss.

Is there any truth to the claim that women live longer than men? If so, is it estrogen?
According to the U.S. Centers for Disease Control (CDC) the average man will live to age 76, while the average woman in America will live to 81. We saw this graph in the Prologue to this book. Pay attention to the difference between females and males. The lines are parallel, but distinctly different over the past 21 years.

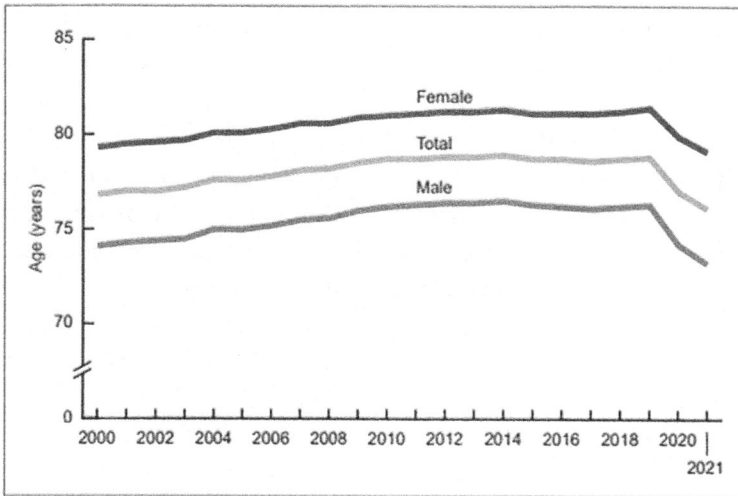

NOTES: Estimates are based on provisional data for 2021. Provisional data are subject to change as additional data are received. Estimates for 2000–2020 are based on final data.
SOURCE: National Center for Health Statistics, National Vital Statistics System, Mortality.

It has been unclear why this difference occurs. At the 2018 North American Menopause Society Annual Meeting, Elissa Epel, Ph.D., described her work looking at the effects of sex hormones, especially estrogen, on the length of telomeres, which, as we stated earlier, protects the endcaps of the DNA. She suggested that estrogen exposure increases the activity of telomerase, the enzyme that can protect and elongate telomeres. She was reluctant to say that all the difference was attributable to estrogen, as other effects such as managing stress, exercising regularly, eating healthy, and getting adequate sleep can also increase telomerase activity.

Paganini-Hill et al. (2018) published an observational study looking at residents of a California retirement community starting in the early 1980s. Their conclusion was that users of estrogen over that time had an age-adjusted mortality that was better than the non-estrogen users by 3.6 years.

Many doctors are concerned about the potential side effects of estrogen therapy in postmenopausal women. One study showed that it reduced the incidence of heart disease in women who took estrogen. Another important study, entitled the Woman's Health Initiative in 2002, suggested that participants who received hormone replacement therapy had an increased risk of breast cancer with no benefit to prevent heart disease. A study by Hodis et al. (2016) showed that women who started hormone therapy within six years of menopause had less atherosclerotic heart disease, but no effect was seen in women who started the estrogen therapy more than 10 years after menopause. He feels that hormone replacement therapy for women has been given a bad image and that proper intervention will prevent problems later.

Proper prospective studies have not been done to answer the question about increasing longevity in women who take estrogen therapy (or even estrogen-progesterone therapy) for that reason. This is something that you should discuss with your health care provider. If you are leaning toward that and your provider is not knowledgeable about the risks and benefits of estrogen therapy, then consider consulting with a specialist in menopause. You might even be able to arrange telehealth visits that way.

If you decide to use estrogen, should you use conjugated estrogen, synthetic estrogen, or bioidentical estrogen? Again, there are strong feelings toward one or the other, but the answers are still not known as to which type of replacement and which dose is the best. Bioidentical hormones refer to hormones that are exactly the same in structure and function as those produced by the human body. They are usually derived from plant or animal tissues and are modified in a laboratory until they are exactly the same as the naturally occurring human hormones. The word "natural" is often misused as one of the most common estrogen replacement medications is Premarin which is derived from the urine of pregnant horses. Cleveland Clinic, in their website, clevelandclinic.com, reviews all the options available. Some prescription forms of bioidentical hormones are premade by drug companies. The U.S. Food and Drug Administration (FDA) has actually approved certain types of bioidentical hormones. Other forms of these are still available, but available only in a laboratory that will custom-make the specific hormone or hormone combination requested by a health care provider. Compounded bioidentical hormones are advertised as being a safer, more effective, natural, and individualized alternative to conventional hormone therapy. However, those claims have yet to be supported by any research. Bioidentical hormones still have the same potential side effects of any type of hormone replacement, including blood clotting disorders, heart disease, breast cancer, or stroke. It is stated that approximately 2.5 million women in the United States over the age of 40 use bioidentical hormones. They come in many forms, including as pills, patches, creams, gels, injections, and even implanted pellets. Some health care providers will attempt to regulate the dosage by serially monitoring blood, urine, or saliva to measure hormone levels. This approach is still unsubstantiated, although theoretically it makes sense. This is a complicated area, and use of any type of estrogen therapy for whatever reason should be discussed at length by the health care provider who will be following you prospectively. Again, we do not have any data to support the use of estrogen to promote longevity.

Dr. Altman has reviewed issues with women as they age. What about age-related changes in sexual performance in men?

Kuzmarov and Bain (2009) reviewed sexuality in the aging couple and wrote specifically about issues with men. The normal male sexual response cycle (Masters & Johnson, 1970) consists of a period of excitement followed by a plateau period, an orgasmic phase, a resolution, and a refractory period. With aging, it is natural for changes to occur. For some men, these changes can lead to distress unless they are made aware of them. These include reductions in spontaneous and early-morning erections, loss of rigidity in the erection and quicker detumescence, reduction in pre-ejaculatory sensation, reduced volume and force of the ejaculate, and reduced need to ejaculate. For some men, other causes may exist, other than just aging. These include lifestyle factors and psychosocial and even psychiatric conditions such as depression, all of which are very prevalent in aging men. Each of these conditions can also lead to erectile dysfunction. There is also a condition called the "Widower's Syndrome," which some men may experience with the resumption of sexual activities after a period of celibacy. When a man has had the same sexual partner for many years, he may enter a new relationship with some trepidation, which, by itself, causes "performance anxiety," which might lead to erectile dysfunction by itself. This performance anxiety (worry about whether he will be able to achieve or maintain his erection) is frequently involved with early signs of erectile dysfunction and may lead to the future inability of achieving any erection at all.

For some men, there are treatments available. It has been shown (Stanworth & Jones, 2006) that testosterone levels decline with age, and testosterone deficiency symptoms can include loss of libido, fatigue, progressive decrease in muscle mass, erectile dysfunction, and depression. Testosterone (by injection, transdermal cream, or oral route) is available for men who have a measured deficiency of testosterone. This diagnosis is often difficult, however, and one that should be confirmed by an endocrinologist or urologist who is used to working with these conditions and knows how to monitor treatment and recognize potential complications. The diagnosis of "testosterone deficiency syndrome" is complicated by the fact that testosterone levels naturally decline with age, so what's "abnormal" is often the decision of the clinician.

Another therapy specifically for erectile dysfunction is the use of phosphodiesterase type 5 inhibitors (PDE-5i's). These medications improve erections in over 50% of men. The use of PDE-5i's has changed the profile of sexual functioning in aging men, offering them the ability to develop erections when they previously could not. The medications currently available are sildenafil (Viagra), tadalafil (Cialis), vardenafil (Levitra), and avanafil (Stendia). The use of these medications needs to be discussed with your health care provider.

We still have not answered the question, "Does having sex regularly contribute to longevity?"

Here is evidence.

There have been reviews discussing "the prescription for a longer life: more sex" (Castleman, 2017). He recommends the standard prescriptions for longevity: eat healthy, exercise daily, don't smoke, get at least 7 hours of sleep each night, don't abuse alcohol or other drugs, and cultivate emotional closeness with friends and family. He also recommends "make love regularly." A study from Wales (Davey-Smith *et al.*, 1997) followed 918 reasonably healthy male residents of the Welsh village, Caerphilly, who were in the age range of 45 to 59 when the study began (1979–1983). When the scientists returned ten years later, 150 had died—67 from cardiac disease and 83 from other causes. They correlated the men's sexual frequency as reported in the original survey with their death or survival ten years later. Compared with men who had sex just once a month, those who reported having it twice a week had only half the death rate. For the entire group, as an individual's sexual frequency increased, his risk of death decreased. The researchers were careful to compare weight, smoking history, blood pressure, and heart disease between the people who were more sexually active and those who were less active and found no difference.

Another study showed that greater sexual frequency is associated with a healthier, longer life. Swedish researchers (Persson, 1981) studied 392 elderly residents of Gothenburg (166 men, 226 women) in the age range of 70 to 75 years. There was a significant association between death and cessation of sexual activity. In another study, researchers compared the sex lives of 100 women who'd had heart attacks and 100 who hadn't. Prior to their heart attacks, the women with heart disease had been much less satisfied with their sex lives.

Adaikan (2014) wrote that sexual health is an integral part of general health that influences the well-being and overall quality of life in men and women. He quoted numerous Internet articles that claimed that sex can do wonders for the well-being of people—that it can reduce anxiety, make you happy, sooth your immunity, decrease neuroticism, and even reduce prostate cancer risk. Only some of the claims have any scientific studies to substantiate them. Sexual activity in the marital setting does have more benefits than in other forms of sexual activity, such as commercial sex or illicit sex. Sexual activity resulting in orgasm does release an assortment of beneficial chemicals in the body. Marital sex does help to bond and strengthen relationships as well as increasing self-worth. He claimed that frequent sex can improve sexual performance, or overall quality of life, and may even extend life by years. He further examined all of the age-related decline in estrogen-related effects on the female anatomy, as well as the decline in sexually related activities in a man, possibly related to testosterone decline. Therefore, based on the existing literature evidence, he felt it was difficult to ascertain whether sexual health per se is a contributing factor for longevity as against the general health and availability of a better health care system.

Last, Dr. Altman recently told us about "sex robots." What are these "sex robots"? According to Wikipedia, sex robots or "sexbots" are anthropomorphic robotic sex dolls that have a humanoid form, human-like movement or behavior, and some degree of artificial intelligence. Although elaborately instrumented sex dolls for males have been created by inventors, no fully animated sex robots yet exist. Simple devices have been created which can speak, make facial expressions, respond to touch, and even develop vaginal lubrication (Maras & Shapiro, 2017). Scholars such as Abdollahi et al. (2017) argue that these robots can act as "robot companions" that aid elderly people with dementia or depression. After conducting a study on many elderly patients, they found that elderly individuals were interested in having an intimate robot as their companion and their interest did not decay over time. They further explained that these patients established meaningful rapport with the robot companion and that they greatly valued its presence. With the use of newly developed artificial skin and artificial intelligence, sexbots could become even more human-like than what are available right now. There are, however, many philosophical objections to the development of these sexbots, including the thought that the introduction of such devices would be socially harmful and demeaning to women and children. There is even a company that announced the creation of the first-ever sexbot for women that will have a customizable bionic penis that can increase in size on demand.

Now for our conclusions. Even though the data presented are far from conclusive in demonstrating in a scientific way the beneficial effects on longevity of frequent sex and frequent orgasms, you must keep in mind that it is exceedingly difficult to do such a study with a control group. Everything published based on surveys is purely observational. On the other hand, there are certainly beneficial effects of having frequent sex when we are in our 60s, 70s, and even 80s. No one of our generation will deny the pleasure associated with sex, so "what the heck." Even if you have vaginal dryness (atrophic vaginitis) and need to use vaginal creams and lubricants; even if you have to take medications, like sildenafil (Viagra) to achieve useable erections; even if it takes you longer than it used to get aroused and longer to ejaculate than it used to; even if it is impossible for you to ejaculate more than once each day and often less than two times a week—it doesn't matter. Enjoy the sex and tell yourself—it feels good, it is good for you, and it might make you live longer as a result. No one will argue with you. Just remember, we only review the science for you and offer suggestions.

We will end our thoughts as follows: Nike (the athletic shoes and sporting goods manufacturer) uses a tagline to promote its sneakers: "Just do it."

We say, "If you have the desire for sex and the ability to perform, just do it when you can. Sex is good for you—and it just might prolong your life."

Role of the Microbiome in Health

When the two of us were starting our professional careers in the late 1970s, the world did not know much about the bacteria in our bodies. We were taught that there are bacteria on our skin, so surgeons need to scrub their hands with surgical soap and wear gloves in the operating room to prevent infections, and that there were bacteria living through our intestines. We were taught that some people who suffered from chronic constipation and/or diarrhea associated often with abdominal cramps were labeled as having "spastic colon" (now called "irritable bowel syndrome") and treatment was directed with antispasmodic medications. We have come a long way in the past 20 years. We now know that there are living organisms all throughout our bodies. These include bacteria, fungi, and viruses, all with their own DNA. As a group they are called the "microbiome." At first, it sounds terrible that there are all those organisms on or in our bodies. We naturally assume that colonization of our body with bacteria, fungi, or viruses would be harmful and potentially lethal. However, it is just the opposite. These organisms protect us against dangerous pathogens (things that can hurt us), help our immune system develop and work properly, enable us to digest the food we eat, and maybe even serve as a source of messages sent to the rest of our bodies (like hormones, cytokines, and neurotransmitters). Bacteria are found on our skin and in our saliva, ileum (small intestine), duodenum, jejunum, dental plaques, and especially in our colons (large intestine). In fact, the majority of the bacteria in our bodies are found in our colons. Estimates have been made as to how many such organisms we have in our bodies. It is only a calculated guess (Sender *et al.*, 2016), but the frequently used number is 39 trillion (3.9×10^{13}). It is said that there are 3×10^{13} cells in our body, which means that there may be more organisms than cells in our bodies. Taking these observations a bit further, perhaps we are not a single living creature, but we are sharing our bodies with all of those organisms, each of which serve a purpose. In a sense, we are a large symbiotic creature.

It is thought that each person has a unique network of microbes, all of which first colonize a baby when the baby passes through the mother's birth canal or when the baby is breastfed. It is important for life that the newborn baby receives exposure to those bacteria as they become very important in nutrition and growth. Babies tend to have the same microbiome as their mothers, but exposure to other experiences can change their microbiome. These include diet and environment. These environmental exposures may actually be harmful in certain cases.

As the baby grows up, things within the microbiome change. Most of the time, there is a symbiotic relationship (both the microbiome and the body benefit). Pathogenetic (disease-causing) bacteria that are kept in check by the usual growth of bacteria. Often there can be a challenge to the body. This might be a radical change in diet, exposure to an infectious agent, and especially when antibiotics are given for a long time. There is a term called "dysbiosis," which refers to a disruption of the normal symbiosis. This can make the body more susceptible to disease (Harvard Health Publishing, 2021).

It is thought that the microbiome contributes to the immune system, breaks down potentially toxic food, and synthesizes certain vitamins and amino acids. These include the B vitamins and Vitamin K. The key enzymes needed to form Vitamin B12 are only found in bacteria, not in plants and animals.

Certain foods, like table sugar (which we do not recommend) and the lactose found in milk, are absorbed in the first part of the intestine. More complex carbohydrates like starches and fibers are not easily digested and travel down to the colon. In the colon are billions of bacteria that help break down those starches using the digestive enzymes of the bacteria. It is thought that this process of fermentation (breaking down of larger substances by bacteria, yeast, or other microorganisms) breaks down otherwise indigestible fibers and causes the production of what are called short-chain fatty acids (SCFA). The SCFAs, the main metabolites produced in the colon by bacterial fermentation of dietary fibers and resistant starch, are speculated to play a key role in neuro-immuno-endocrine regulation. However, the underlying mechanisms through which SCFAs might influence brain physiology and behavior have not been fully elucidated. The same SCFA can be used by the body as a source of nutrition, but they may also play a role in muscle function and in the prevention of certain chronic diseases, including bowel disorders. Clinical studies have also shown that SCFA may be useful in the treatment of ulcerative colitis, regional enteritis, and antibiotic-associated diarrhea.

The microbiome of a healthy person will also provide protection from pathogenic organisms that enter the body through eating or drinking contaminated food or water.

There is a network of cellular and chemical signaling between the gut and the nervous system. (Terry & Margolis, 2017). There is a direct correlation between poor gut microbiome compositions and neuromuscular conditions ranging from Parkinson's disease, to anxiety, depression, irritable bowel syndrome, inflammatory bowel disease, and possibly even autism (Kohn, 2015). As Jameson et al. (2020) suggested, there is strong evidence pointing to select members of the microbiome displaying the ability to synthesize and/or regulate various neurochemicals. If that is true, can you imagine how many people might have suffered mental health concerns because of the lack of healthy bacteria in their intestines? Serotonin, possibly the mediator of mental and emotional stability, is a hormone that creates signaling pathways for balanced physiology and psychology, sensory processing, cognitive control, emotional regulation, autonomic response, and even motor activity. Although serotonin is considered a "brain hormone," 90% of the serotonin in the body is synthesized in the intestine (Terry & Margolis, 2017). These were also the conclusions of Grenham et al. (2011), Clemente et al. (2012), and Carpenter (2012).

Colonized microbial communities are responsible for the production of this neurotransmitter. A 2001 study (Mossner et al., 2001) revealed immune signaling and serotonin. There is a link between neuronal signaling and immune response establishing a well-defined neuroimmune communication network throughout the body. As a matter of fact, at least one study showed that serotonin lets the T cells know when there is cancer present so that the immune system can begin resisting its growth (Karmakar & Lal, 2021).

You should now begin to understand that the microbiome can be thought of as an organ in itself, contributing in many ways to the health and well-being of the human body.

For the record, the names of the families of bacteria usually found in the human colon include *Prevotella, Ruminococcus, Bacteroides*, and *Firmicutes*. Because of the very low oxygen environment in the colon, there is also found what is called "anaerobic" bacteria (able to survive in very low or no oxygen content). These include *Peptostreptococcus, Bifidobacterium, Lactobacillus*, and *Clostridium*. Those are the microbes that are thought to prevent the overgrowth of harmful bacteria by competing for nutrients and attaching to certain sites of the lining of the colon.

Now we need to explore what happens when the normal microbiome gets disrupted. A major cause of this disruption is the extensive use of antibiotics in our society and the unexpected consequences. Antibiotics have saved millions of lives since their inception. Starting in the 1940s, penicillin quickly became the grandad of all antibiotics and helped to win the war against fatal bacterial infections. This category of drugs were initially so successful that they became universally embraced by physicians, and they were used not only in a conservative way but were also overused and applied for too long. These antibiotics are different from other pharmaceuticals that not only affect the individual to whom they are applied but also other life forms they interact with. Secreted from our bodies, these antibiotics may even get into the aquafer and widely destroy the naturally occurring microbes that are in soil and water. This triggers an ecosystem imbalance that moves up the chain and ironically once again affects humans. There is an ever-growing catalog of studies that focus on the ill-effects that antibiotics have on human health. Obesity, type I and type II diabetes, inflammatory bowel disease, celiac disease, allergies, and asthma are among the top modalities that may be precipitated by antibiotic overuse (Blaser, 2016). When an antibiotic is ingested, it goes through the villi of the small intestine creating cell damage that results in immune cell activation in the production of antimicrobial peptides. This puts into play a number of biochemical actions resulting in a gut–immune imbalance. Inflammation is provoked by this process that significantly increases the odds of contracting some sort of disease. Nearly half of antibiotics are used for raising animals which most of the world consumes as food. As much as 87% of these drugs that are applied on these victimized animals are either never, or very rarely, used in human medicine. For this reason, it bombards the human body with anti-life medicines resulting in antibiotic resistance. There is a bottom line in this discussion: "healthy gut bacteria allow all systems and all organs to function effectively and successfully."

Other types of stress to the microbiome could cause the same dysbiosis. Unfortunately, we do not know all of them. It could be the types of foods we consume, the herbicides and pesticides used to grow food, the chemicals used in food processing, and possibly genetically modified organisms (GMO). Our food and water intake is thought to be the most significant cause of the dysbiosis and the factors that are the most under our own control.

Are there any conditions in which a health care provider might want to remove certain bacterial flora in the microbiome and replace them with different ones? This is the so-called fecal microbial transplant. A "fecal transplant" is a procedure that removes the intestinal content including the bacteria with a strong "bowel prep" for a patient's colon and replaces that with the stool from a healthy person or from a "bank" of stools from normal people without gastrointestinal conditions. A doctor may call it "bacteriotherapy." Fecal transplantation has been used for more than 100 years by veterinarians to treat horses with uncontrollable diarrhea. It has been used in humans since 1958. Because of the implication, this procedure has been studied for the following conditions:

- Ulcerative colitis (Lopetuso *et al.*, 2020)
- Crohn's disease (Gutin *et al.,* 2019)
- Cirrhosis (Hassouneh & Bajaj, 2021)
- Multiple sclerosis (Makkawi *et al.,* 2018)
- Depression (Meyyappan *et al.,* 2020)
- Obesity (Napolitano & Covasa, 2020)
- Food allergies (Lee *et al.*, 2020)
- Painful diabetic neuropathy (Cai *et al.,* 2018)

Each of the above conditions has been treated with fecal transplantation, all with mixed results. Fecal transplants do show a lot of promise as treatments for ulcerative colitis (UC), which is often associated with an unhealthy mix of gut bacteria. In one study, people with UC received a fecal transplant that used "poop" mixed from two donors. Some saw improved symptoms and lower inflammation only a month later, and 15% of patients went into remission. There is some evidence that donor "matching" can improve the chance of success for people with UC. In addition, it seems that family members often make better donors than those chosen at random. Sibling donors seem to do better than parent or child donors, possibly because they tend to be closer in age. More research is needed to learn why fecal transplants work for some people with UC but not for others. The same is true for all the other above medical conditions. The promise seems wonderful, but, so far, the results have not been universally successful.

These studies are all significant in another way. Some people who apparently have an unhealthy microbiome will improve their symptoms with new intestinal bacteria. This observation is extremely important, and ongoing research may provide the answers as to which patients will benefit the most and what type of feces should be used to improve their disease.

There is one condition, on the other hand, which has been studied extensively, and the use of fecal transplants has been extremely successful. Some people suffer from recurrent *Clostridium difficile* infection. This is thought to be a result of overgrowth of those bacteria, as a result of patients who receive antibiotics. In fact, the infection at one time was called "*Clostridial* colitis." It presents with uncontrollable diarrhea. Even though most patients who suffer from this condition do respond to treatment with a different combination of antibiotics, some people do not and suffer from recurrent severe diarrhea. This condition occurs because antibiotics perturb patients' intestinal microbiome (Brandt, 2012). With appropriate treatment including a special antibiotic, the condition is cured in 90% or so of patients with *Clostridial* colitis. In 10% it does not. For these 10%, the community of living organisms in the intestine will no longer be able to protect the host against *C. difficile* infection. By reintroducing a healthy diversity of bacteria, fecal transplantation can reestablish colonization resistance to prevent *C. difficile* from becoming a dominant organism in the environment of the gut.

So, what can we do to nurture or enhance our microbiome to make us have healthier lives and live longer?

William Bulsiewicz, M.D., a gastroenterologist in South Carolina, stated that the single greatest predictor of a healthy gut is the diversity of plants one consumes. Tomova *et al*. (2019) reported that a plant-based diet fosters a greater microbial diversity. A positive association between local bacterial richness and long-term plant-based intake confirmed its benefit for biological and psychological well-being. Most important was the finding that uncooked and unprocessed enzymes in fiber-rich plant foods acted as the most beneficial fuel for healthy fauna/flora. There are plant metabolites, called "polyphenols," that increase two of the most important gut bacteria that provide anti-pathogenic and anti-inflammatory effects along with cardiovascular protection. Once you cook the vegetable, these benefits are gone. With the elimination of animal-based foods and the movement toward plant-based eating, you naturally gravitate to consuming high-quality choices such as organic vegetables, sprouts, raw nuts, and seeds. Contained within such foods are polyunsaturated fats that increase beneficial bacterial ratios.

It should be obvious now that the intestinal bacteria (our own unique microbiome) need to be nurtured and cared for properly. We should strive toward a plant-based diet, consuming as many fresh organically grown vegetables as we can. We should limit the use of all chemicals that could interfere with our flora, especially antibiotics. We should never ask our health care provider to prescribe antibiotics for us for what is obviously a common cold, most certainly caused by a virus that never responds to antibiotics. We should discuss with our health care provider which antibiotic will be prescribed, making sure that the least broad-spectrum antibiotic be used. The stronger the antibiotic, the more intestinal bacteria are disturbed. Also, the use of an antibiotic should be as short a term as possible to cause the least damage and allow the microbiome to recover.

Should we all take "probiotics" either routinely or during or immediately after a prescribed course of antibiotic therapy or use them to just stay healthy?

Probiotics are marketed aggressively in health-food stores. Unfortunately, there are so many different products out there, all of which claim to have miraculous results in promoting intestinal health. Probiotics are substances that contain live bacteria. There are some food products that are promoted as having probiotics. Yogurt is the most common type of food, but cheese, kefir, kimchi, and sauerkraut all have probiotics as well. We are not proponents of yogurt, cheese, and kefir because they contain milk products. In addition, one can find many different types and brands of probiotics. Some are on the shelf. Some are kept in the refrigerator; some are frozen.

Here is a picture taken in a grocery store displaying many different types. Who knows what to take?

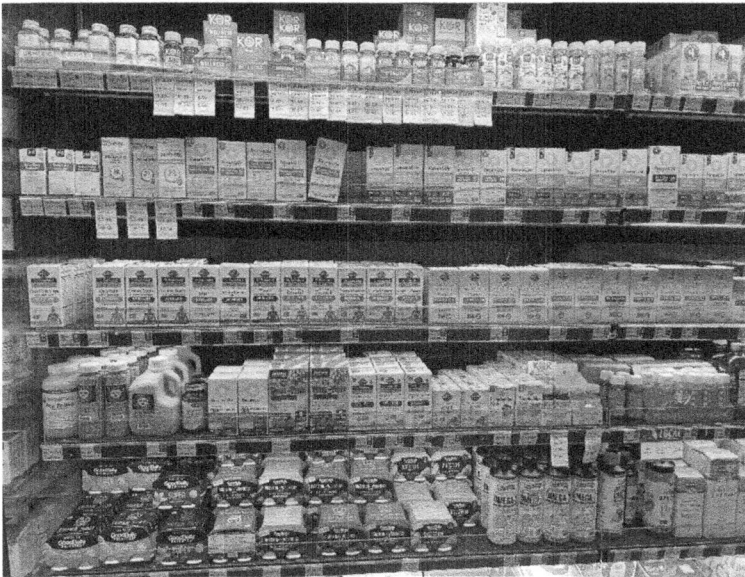

It is easy now to see why the probiotic supplement sales exceeded $35 billion in 2015 with the projected amount of $64 billion occurring in 2024. Whether you believe these intestinal health claims or whether you think that probiotics are a snake oil scam, they still represent a multibillion-dollar industry.

Dr. Allan Walker, Professor of Nutrition at the Harvard T.H. Chan School of Public Health, believes that taking probiotics might be most effective in the very young and very old individuals after a course of antibiotics. He feels that the normal microbes in the colon may not be as robust as during the middle years of life. Another potential use is in reducing the severity of diarrhea after exposure to certain antibiotics.

Because probiotics fall under the category of food supplements, and not food, they are not regulated by the Food and Drug Administration agency in the United States. That means the manufacturer does not have to adhere to rigorous quality standards. So, any given probiotic may not have the activity it claims or even have bacteria that are alive.

What about "prebiotics"? Prebiotics are foods and supplements that will support the production of SFCA. They feed our beneficial microbiome. Some of the specific foods that serve that purpose are garlic, onions, leeks, asparagus, Jerusalem artichokes, dandelion greens, bananas, and seaweed. Also, fruits, vegetables, beans, whole grains (wheat, oats, and barley) are all good sources of prebiotic fibers. These are a major part of a plant-based diet. As a word of caution, if any of you make the decision to start a program by eating all of these products, you might suddenly have extreme flatulence (gas) and bloating until your intestines get used to the new diet. It is best to introduce those items slowly.

Other nutritionists recommend fermented food on a regular basis. In addition to yogurt, these include kefir, sauerkraut, kimchi, miso, pickled vegetables, rejuvelac, tempeh, and kombucha.

A more scientific approach to understand what our microbiome is composed of would be to find a laboratory that will culture a stool sample, maybe obtained during a colonoscopy. The laboratory would identify and quantitate the specific bacteria and fungi that live there to see if your results are considered normal compared to others who have no medical problems or if the composition is consistent with that seen in other people with similar symptoms or disease. A Google search generated over ten such companies, all of whom will do the work for you at a cost but will also try to sell you something to fill in what is missing. Until norms are established for both healthy persons and diseased persons, we are not sure if that approach even works. We always caution our patients and guests away from anything that sounds like profiteering.

With all this information, what should a person do right now? We hope you see that your microbiome is just as important as any other part of your body and, in itself, may contribute immensely toward disease prevention and longevity. One day we may know the reasons why our microbiome depends upon a balanced intestinal flora and a high-greens diet. Our message to you is that if you are looking for a reason to change to a plant-based diet, this may be that reason. If this way of eating is new to you, consider creating a realistic plan to remove health-destructive foods and systematically replace them with health-restorative choices.

Will improving your microbiome help you to live longer? At this time, no one knows for sure. Following our suggestions might make a difference. Again, it is your choice.

CHAPTER 8

Can Stem Cells Help?

According to the Mayo Clinic, stem cells are the body's raw materials—cells from which all other cells with specialized functions are generated. Under certain conditions, either in the body, or in the laboratory, stem cells will divide to form more cells called "daughter cells." These daughter calls will become either new stem cells or specialized cells that can become bone cells, heart muscle cells, brain cells, or blood cells. No other cells in the body have the ability to generate new cell types.

It is thought that human beings originate from a total-potential stem cell, the fertilized egg. After birth, the proliferation and differentiation of these stem cells contribute to the development and maturation of individual tissues and organs. After maturation, aging is a phase of the life process; the stem cells within the individual's tissues ensure the metabolism of different cells and tissues. An example of this process are the cells that make up the blood cells in the bone marrow, which ensure there are still enough red blood cells to transport oxygen after a single RBC has completed its 120-day physiological lifecycle.

Other examples of the aging process occur in the intestinal and kidney cells. After pathological damage and necrosis occurs, there will be regenerative cells that continue to maintain the integrity of the structure and function of the intestine and the kidneys. The role of stem cells in the regeneration and repair of tissues and organs is not only due to the ability of proliferation and differentiation of stem cells but also due to the secretion function of stem cells, which secrete various growth factors and cytokines to regulate the tissue microenvironment. In other words, these same stem cells can control their own life by communication through biological messages.

Researchers in the field are working with stem cells in an effort to accomplish the following:

- Increase the understanding of how diseases occur.
- Generate healthy cells to replace cells affected by disease.

The hope is that one day doctors may have available specific therapies for those people, for example, those who have had such diverse conditions as spinal cord injuries; type 1 diabetes; neurological conditions, such as Amyotrophic Lateral Sclerosis (ALS), Parkinson's disease, and Alzheimer's disease; heart diseases and stroke; burns; and cancer. At the present time, active research is going on in each of these areas, with no results to share, as yet.

Stem cells can be found or obtained from several sources:

- Embryonic stem cells
  - These stem cells come from embryos that are 3 to 5 days old. An embryo is the early stage of development of a multicellular organism. It occurs shortly after fertilization. These cells can divide into more stem cells or to become any cell in the body if we are talking about human cells. This versatility allows the embryonic stem cells to be used to repair or regenerate diseased tissue or organs.
- Adult stem cells
  - These types of stem cells can be found in small numbers in most adult tissues, especially in the bone marrow (the place where blood cells are created) or in fat. It is thought that these adult stem cells have a more limited ability to give rise to various cells of the body. It is hoped that one day adult stem cells may be able to be manipulated into various types of cells. Perhaps one day, bone marrow stem cells may be able to create heart muscle or neurological cells.
- Adult cells altered to have properties of embryonic stem cells
  - Scientists are currently working to try to transform adult stem cells into more primitive stem cells using genetic reprogramming. Messages would be sent to the genes within these cells to program them to function like embryonic stem cells.
- Perinatal stem cells
  - Stem cells have been found in amniotic fluid (the fluid that helps to nurture a growing baby inside the mother's womb) and in the umbilical cord (the organ that nurtures the growing baby). These stem cells have the potential to become more specialized cells.

Stem cell therapy has been successfully used in what is called "bone marrow transplants." This type of therapy has been most effective to replace cells damaged by chemotherapy or a disease itself. These stem cell transplants

have been successfully used to fight some forms of cancer, as well as leuke-
mia, lymphoma, and multiple myeloma, among other blood disorders. These
transplants use adult stem cells or umbilical cord blood. Research is ongoing
in the use of stem cells in treating other conditions such as refractory congestive heart failure.

One of the potential problems in using stem cells is to make sure that
the stem cells will actually become the specific cell types desired. There
are many other potential problems, including a situation in which the recipient's body attacks the stem cells as foreign invaders or the stem cells
just do not function as expected or the newly transplanted or implanted
stem cells attack its host (or recipient) in what is called "Graft vs. Host
Disease."

In addition, there is a major controversy about where to obtain these
stem cells. The stem cells that seem to have the most potential to be directed into becoming specific cells in the body are those that are obtained
from early-stage embryos. These are usually obtained at an IVF (in vitro fertilization) lab. Because the human embryonic stem cells are extracted from
human embryos, several ethical issues are raised. The National Institutes
of Health (NIH) created specific guidelines for human stem cell research
in 2009. These guidelines define embryonic stem cells and how they can
be used in research. They also state that the embryos created in an IVF
lab can be used only when the embryo is no longer needed. That means
that a woman has many eggs extracted (or were previously extracted and
frozen), and those eggs have been fertilized by male sperm cells in a so-
called test tube. At the time of the procedure many such fertilized eggs are
created. Usually only one or two of these fertilized eggs are implanted into
a woman's womb. The rest of those unused fertilized eggs theoretically
could be donated with informed consent from the donors. The stem cells
can theoretically live and grow in the laboratory. The ethics of doing this
can create many problems, and the numbers of stem cells available in this
way are greatly limited.

Adult stem cells may not be as versatile as are the embryonic stem
cells. They may not be able to be manipulated to change into other cells,
which limits their usage. Also, theoretically, adult stem cells may contain
environmental toxins. All these issues are currently being worked on, and
there exists some degree of optimism that adult stem cells can one day
be used.

Another area of ongoing research is to create stem cells lines. These
are a group of cells that all come from a single original stem cell and are

grown in a specialized lab. These cells are being programmed only to reproduce, but not to differentiate into, specialized cells. One day, if the cells turn out to be free of genetic defects, they can be programmed to become specific tissue cells when the need arises. This is very interesting work but not universally or clinically available now. If this technique is ever perfected, a scientist could inject these cells into the heart muscle of a person with a failing heart, for example. These are the stem cells that have been programmed to become heart cells. They then contribute to replacing the injured heart muscle. This represents cell transplantation and not organ transplantation.

Still another area of research is called "therapeutic cloning" or "somatic cell nuclear transfer." This is a technique to create stem cells independent of fertilized eggs. In the laboratory, the nucleus is removed from an unfertilized egg. This nucleus contains all the genetic material to create a human. The nucleus of a cell obtained from a donor is also removed and injected into the egg, replacing the nucleus that was removed. If this process, hopefully, works, the new egg is allowed to divide and soon becomes an embryo, creating a line of stem cells that are genetically identical to the donor's cells. If this process works, there might be less rejection during the therapy of transplanting the cells. Up to this point, this therapeutic cloning has not worked in humans, although it has worked in other species.

So, what about aging? Do stem cells have a role in reversing or slowing down the aging process?

Aging can be thought of as a natural phase of the life process, and all creatures obey this rule of nature. Different organs of the body age at different rates. Aging is reflected in structural changes and reduced function of these organs. Among them, the reduction of regeneration and repair capacity is the main feature of aging. As we age, the aging of stem cells in human tissues might be a major cause of the decline in tissue regeneration capacity. Therefore, the elderly's ability to regenerate and repair might be improved by application of advanced stem cell technology.

Stem cells seem to play a crucial role in delaying the aging process. Stem cells, in combination with anti-aging genes, can create a sophisticated shield that supposedly can prevent the effects of aging. Increased wear and tear on the body's natural stem cells increases cellular damage and accelerates the natural process of aging. Some people claim that the introduction of "youthful" stem cells into the human body can rejuvenate existing cells and allow the body to age more gracefully or more slowly and even reverse some effects of the aging process. As we age, our cells lose function and eventually die. When a cell dies, it creates a cascade of events, leading to inflammation and disease that can decrease the human life span.

Rožman (2019) reviewed evidence that delaying and reversing aging in cells is feasible. Epigenetic (nongenetic influences on gene expression) changes drive aging, and a reversal of these changes extends life span. Epigenetic control of gene expression occurs by modification of DNA.

Aging is considered as inevitable changes at different levels of genome (where the DNA is), cell, and organism. From the accumulation of DNA damages to imperfect protein homeostasis, altered cellular communication, and exhaustion of stem cells, aging is a major risk factor for many prevalent diseases, such as cancer, cardiovascular disease, pulmonary disease, diabetes, and neurological disorders. The cells are dynamic systems, which, through a cycle of processes such as replication, growth, and death, could replenish the body's organs and tissues, keeping an entire organism in optimal working order. In many different tissues, adult stem cells theoretically might be behind these processes, replenishing dying cells to maintain normal tissue function and regenerating injured tissues. Therefore, adult stem cells might play a vital role in preventing the aging of organs and tissues and delaying aging.

With current knowledge on stem cells, it is feasible to design and test interventions that delay aging and improve both health and life span. Stem cells, together with anti-aging genes such as α-Klotho (a gene involved in the aging process of mammals), play a crucial role in delaying the aging process. Stem cells in combination with anti-aging genes make a complex and protective shield that stands against the eroding effects of aging. Increased wear and tear of the stem cells, as well as α-Klotho deficiency, is expected to heavily increase cellular damage and accelerate the process of aging. Stem cells in conjugation with anti-aging genes probably receive and neutralize most of the devastating signaling effects that are known to cause premature aging. The shield of stem cells combined with anti-aging genes is a primary target for absorbing the shock of aging. If this shield neutralizes the shocks, it could lead to a youthful state, but if not, it will accelerate the aging journey. Ullah and Sun (2018) suggest that stem cell interventions can increase rejuvenation and keep in balance the expression of anti-aging genes which could delay the aging phenotypes and result in prolonged life span.

Contributing Factors Toward Aging	
Accumulation of toxic metabolites	Impaired Regulation of Reactive Oxygen Species
Inflammation	Impaired Autophagy
Poor Immune System	Hormonal Disorder
Failures in DNA Damage Repair System	Genetic Dysfunction
Exhaustion of Stem Cell Pool	Diseases (heart, kidney, diabetes, cancer, immune disorders, neurological)
Impaired Regeneration	Toxic Metabolites
Epigenetic Alterations	
Senescence	Personal Life Style
Apoptosis	Obesity
Necrosis	Diet and Drinks
Loss of Proliferation and Self Renewal	Stress
Telomere and Genomic Instability	
Stem Cells Depletion	Environmental Stressors
	Radiation
	Pollution

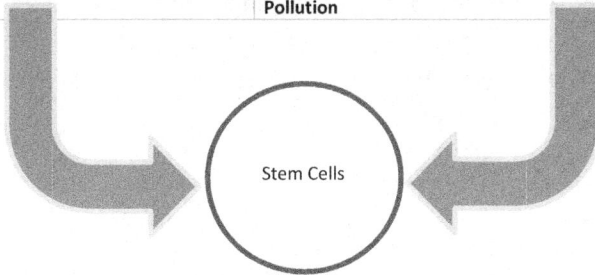

Stem Cells

But do they work, and where can you get "the stuff"? Are stem cells the true "Fountain of Youth"? Here is what we know.

Zhang *et al.* (2017) conducted experiments in which they injected stem cells into the hypothalamus of the brains of mice. They discovered that this process extended the lives by 10% to 15% and slowed the aging process in older mice. Their theory is that these cells release microRNAs which are not involved in protein synthesis but instead play key roles in regulating gene expression. MicroRNAs are packaged inside tiny particles called "exosomes," which hypothalamic stem cells release into the cerebrospinal fluid of mice. However, that type of experiment can obviously not be performed in humans. There are abundant stem cells in the hypothalamus of the human brain in youth, but they are almost all gone by middle age.

No matter what trial is undertaken for observing any modification of human longevity, it is a difficult and long process. It might take many years to see whether there are any differences in people who receive the experimental treatment versus their age-matched controls. Measuring effects on longevity is very difficult to do, but exceptionally so when doing a study using a biological product like stem cells.

In addition, it is hard to do stem cell research in the United States. In 2010, there was a court order on stem cell research. The court order was the outcome of a lawsuit originally filed against the Department of Health and Human Services (HHS) and the National Institutes of Health (NIH) in Bethesda, Maryland, which contended that federal funding for research on human embryonic stem cells was illegal because it requires the destruction of embryos. There has been some activity since that court order, but nothing has been changed to give a go-ahead to research as originally begun.

However, that has not stopped companies from obtaining and dispensing stem cells. A potential patient has to travel out of the country to receive the treatments. Turner and Knoepfler (2016) found that there were 351 businesses operating 570 clinics domestically, and many provide services that claim to treat a wide range of illnesses with a lack of scientific oversight. Here is a map copied from that paper that shows how many clinics there were in the United States in 2016.

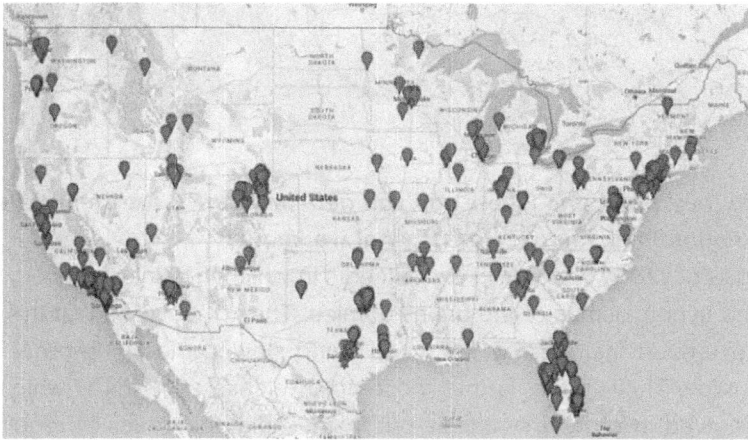

These clinics advertise different stem cell procedures. As much 61% use autologous adipose-derived stem cell–based interventions, 48% market what they describe as autologous stem cells obtained from bone marrow, and 4% market stem cells reportedly obtained from peripheral blood. They market themselves as being able to treat a wide range of disease and injuries, as well as for use in cosmetics, sexual enhancement, orthopedic and sports medicine, neurodegenerative conditions, spinal cord injuries, immunological conditions, pulmonary disorders, ophthalmological diseases and injuries, urological diseases, as well as cosmetic indications. Many of these marketing claims give rise to significant ethical issues given the lack of peer-reviewed evidence that advertised stem cell interventions are safe and efficacious for the treatment of certain diseases. Such promotional claims also generate regulatory concerns due to apparent noncompliance with federal regulations.

The use of stem cells as part of anti-aging also falls into this category of regulatory concern and unproved results. Once companies start to make strong marketing claims offering stem cells for things like ALS, muscular dystrophy, Parkinson's disease, and Alzheimer's disease, there should be concerns on the part of the consumer on whether the company is totally compliant with FDA rules and regulations and even if these companies ever submit their results of their research for peer review.

The prevalence of these advertisements should make us concerned about ethical issues because most of these claims do lack peer-reviewed scientific evidence that the procedures used are safe and, especially, are effective. The FDA has issued a warning about some of the claims. Meanwhile, the International Society for Stem Cell Research released guidelines in 2015 that warned the majority of treatments that these clinics offer are unproven, with "adverse events" frequently reported after these procedures.

If you still want to try stem cell therapy to prolong your life, you might consider the following locations where you can go if you want to try a treatment not available in the United States. We obtained this information from a Google search.

Australia	India
Caribbean Islands	Mexico
China	South Korea
Costa Rica	Thailand

There is even a jargon called "stem cell tourism," in which a patient cannot obtain what he or she wants in the United States and is willing to pay to travel. There are prearranged luxury accommodations while a patient waits while obtaining care at those places.

Let's explore the options available to make you aware of the situation if you decide to take stem cells to prolong your life, despite the lack of published longitudinal studies exploring the use of stem cells.

Cost is an important factor, independent of the travel expenses associated with going to a center, and the accommodations needed while you are there.

- The cost depends upon the following factors:
  - The disease for which stem cell treatment is selected

- The type of stem cells administered
  - Platelet-rich plasma (PRP) injections
  - Birth tissues (umbilical cord blood or amniotic fluid)
  - Fat tissue or bone marrow
- Allogenic culture–expanded stem cell procedure (umbilical cord tissue). This is the most expensive and ranges from $15,000 to $50,000. In addition, these types of cells cannot be used in the United States because they are not authorized according to the FDA. There are studies that suggest growing stem cells in tissue culture will reduce the efficacy of stem cells.

Stem cells are acquired by companies that pay hospitals for donated cord tissue or by doctors who perform fat tissue or bone marrow extractions. The cells are then sent to separate laboratories that specialize in stem cell expansion. These labs usually have very qualified and specialized staff members and are under the strict regulations of the FDA. The cells are then shipped in cryogenic storage overnight around the world to the stem cell clinics. These clinics are staffed with doctors, nurses, and support staff who all play a part in the patient's experience. In every stage of this process, there are heavy costs associated with time and labor, before the patient is ever given treatment. This information was found on the DVCSTEM website (https://www.dvcstem.com/), a company operating out of the Cayman Islands.

In other countries, there is much less regulation to ensure the safety and viability of the cells.

Many people need only one treatment. Some people come back every year for repeat treatments. Medicare does not cover stem cell therapy in the United States or elsewhere.

Here is a partial list of overseas stem cell treatment centers, obtained via a Google Search.

- GIOSTAR in Mexico
- Stem Cell Institute in Panama
- Regenexx in Cayman Islands
- DVC Stem in Grand Cayman
- Okyanos in Grand Bahamas
- Celltex in Mexico

This list may be far from complete because in September 2019, Google banned ads for "unproven or experimental medical techniques such as most stem cell therapy and gene therapy. The treatments, the company says in the statement, can have potentially dangerous health outcomes and have no place on its platform." Unfortunately, that move on the part of Google generated controversy, and there was pressure on Google to make public the process they use to vet ads and decide what standards they use for determining the effectiveness of a specific treatment. The International Society for Stem Cell Research welcomed Google's decision. The ISSCR felt that selling treatments before well-regulated clinical trials have been done and could undermine the development of new legitimate therapies.

Despite these types of concerns (where the stem cells come from and whether their use actually does anything), it is easy to see how less scrupulous companies can exploit the allure of stem cells that seem to provide a magical elixir, the "Fountain of Youth." There are legitimate scientists who are optimistic that one day humans can live forever. Unfortunately, that claim is many years away. Appropriate stem cell therapy could very well be a part of that concept.

Just to tempt you about what is going on in the research world, Professor Ilaria Bellantuono working at the Healthy Lifespan Institute at the University of Sheffield Medical School, is studying "senolytics." This is a type of medication that could kill off our aging cells, the so-called zombie cells that accumulate in tissues as we age and can cause chronic inflammation. She feels that her data in animal models indicate that senolytics are able to delay the onset and reduce the severity of multiple diseases at the same time, including osteoarthritis, osteoporosis, cardiovascular disease, Alzheimer's disease, Parkinson's disease, and diabetes. She feels that this type of treatment could actually be more cost effective than stem cell therapy and the status quo of older patients taking multiple pills for multiple diseases which may not interact well with each other. This could become another approach to that "Fountain of Youth" (see Chapter 13.)

Now, if you are determined that you want to take stem cells to prevent your body from aging, and you can afford the cost of going overseas for an unapproved stem cell treatment, what side effects might occur? (These are actually side effects described by WebMD on their website webmd.com)

- Fatigue and weakness
- Flu-like symptoms
- Nausea
- Altered sense of taste or smell

Other side effects are associated with the chemotherapy directed against the primary disease that you are treating.

One specific use of stem cells that has received much publicity lately through intensive marketing is the use of anti-aging skin products that contain stem cells. Over the past few years, more and more facial creams have been introduced into the U.S. markets claiming to minimize the appearance of wrinkles and to slow down, or even reverse, the course of aging. Under the guise of terms like "scientifically engineered," these creams claim to harness the power of stem cells or stem cell extracts. Some companies have even coined a new word, "cosmeceuticals," to give the impression that the product has a drug-like benefit. An article in *Boston* magazine in 2013 concluded: "The term 'cosmeceuticals' is not recognized by the U.S. Food and Drug Administration and thus not subject to its regulatory scope. What this means is that not one of these products is required to prove the validity of the science it preaches for its products. To date, none of these companies have published any significant data in the literature that proves their effectiveness. Furthermore, no stem cells could even survive long term embedded in a cream, let alone be guaranteed to work on all individuals (your body would be more likely to reject foreign cells)."

Deciding to take stem cells in 2023 without any guarantee of improving longevity is up to the individual person and his or her family. It is possible that, one day, scientists will have this all figured out and will understand exactly what our own aging stem cells can no longer do and how or when they will need to be replaced. We would even have an accepted protocol in place for all to follow, including knowing the best source of obtaining the stem cells to use. In addition, having enough data regarding efficacy and side effects and having in place a more ethically accepted way to harvest stem cells should be the type of information the FDA will need to approve the treatment. Once that occurs, the procedure could be done in the United States, with proper medical backup on site. Once all those concerns are resolved, Medicare might then cover the treatments, especially if the treatments will prevent or reverse degenerative diseases, especially those associated with expensive long-term care.

As in other chapters of our book, we want to present information to you so that you can decide whether this treatment is for you. Maybe, one day, when we all have achieved that 120-year-old mark, we might have been given stem cell treatment or senolytics (see Chapter 12) in our local hospitals or medical centers and be happy that the treatment was so effective. We are just not there yet.

CHAPTER 9

Health Care and Insurance

Baby Boomers usually start to worry about their health insurance when they pass their 60th birthday and know that they will have some choices to make once they reach age 65. Prior to that time, they are usually covered by a health insurance plan provided, and often paid for, by their employer, and may even be required to contribute to the monthly premiums themselves. Although health insurance, by itself, does not contribute to longevity, we thought it would be important to include a discussion on health insurance for Baby Boomers.

Prior to age 65, people either have a health insurance policy or have no insurance and pay privately for all their health-related expenses. That includes doctor visits, urgent care center visits, emergency room visits, laboratory and other diagnostic tests, surgery, anesthesia-related expenses, and, of course, medications and hospitalizations.

According to Statista Research Department, in October 2021, 91.4% of people in the United States were covered by some type of health insurance. As much as 50.3% received insurance through their employer and 39.5% had public health insurance, most of whom have Medicare or Medicaid. It could be a Preferred Provider Organization (PPO), or it could be a Health Maintenance Organization (HMO). The amount of the premium paid by the employer varies tremendously. Some employers will cover family insurance of the employee; others require the employee to pay for that coverage separately. Some people elect ObamaCare, which is similar to a PPO available to people who do not have employer-sponsored plans.

Most people over age 65 elect to enroll in the Medicare program. Medicare is a federal health insurance program for those who are 65 years old or older, although certain people with disabilities and people who have end-stage renal (kidney) disease (ESRD) are also eligible. You may sign up for Medicare three months before you turn 65. When you first enroll, you will receive the original Medicare, unless you chose to enroll in a Medicare advantage plan (HMO).

Traditional Medicare has several parts (www.medicare.gov).

Part A (Hospital Insurance) helps cover inpatient care in hospitals, skilled nursing facility care, hospice care, and homecare. Please note that it "helps," but does not always pay all the costs.

Part B (Medical Insurance) helps cover:

- Services from doctors and other health care providers
- Outpatient care
- Home health care
- Durable medical equipment (like wheelchairs, walkers, hospital beds, and other equipment)
- Some preventive services (like screenings, shots, or vaccines, and yearly wellness visits).

Part D (Drug Coverage) helps cover the cost of prescription drugs (including many recommended shots or vaccines.) You can opt to join a Medicare drug plan in addition to Original Medicare, or you get it by joining a Medicare Advantage Plan with drug coverage. Plans that offer Medicare drug coverage are run by private insurance companies that follow rules set by Medicare.

Medicare Supplemental Insurance (Medigap) is extra insurance you can buy from a private company that helps pay your share of costs in Original Medicare. Policies are standardized, and, in most states, are named by letters, like Plan G or Plan K. The benefits in each lettered plan are the same, no matter which insurance company sells it.

The website www.medicare.gov contains the following table that explains some of the differences between Original Medicare and Medicare Advantage (also known as Part C).

Original Medicare	Medicare Advantage (Part C)
- Original Medicare includes Part A and Part B. - You can join a separate Medicare drug plan to get Medicare Drug Coverage (Part D). - You can use any doctor or hospital that takes Medicare, anywhere in the United States.	- Medicare Advantage is a Medicare-approved plan from a private company that offers an alternative to Original Medicare for your health and drug coverage. These "bundled" plans include Part A, Part B, and usually Part D.

Original Medicare	Medicare Advantage (Part C)
▪ To help pay your out-of-pocket costs in Original Medicare (like your 20% coinsurance), you can also buy supplemental coverage, like Medicare Supplement Insurance (Medigap), or have coverage from a former employer or union, or Medicaid.	▪ In most cases, you will need to use doctors who are in the plan's network. ▪ Plans may have lower out-of-pocket costs than Original Medicare. ▪ Plans may offer some extra benefits that Original Medicare does not cover—like vision, hearing, and dental services.

Other differences to consider:

Doctor and Hospital Choice

Original Medicare	Medicare Advantage (Part C)
You can go to **any doctor or hospital that takes Medicare, anywhere in the United States.**	In many cases, you'll need to only use **doctors and other providers who are in the plan's network** (for nonemergency care). Some plans offer nonemergency coverage out of network, but typically at a higher cost.
In most cases, you **don't need** a referral to see a specialist.	You **may need** to get a referral to see a specialist.

Cost

Original Medicare	Medicare Advantage (Part C)
For Part B-covered services, **you usually pay 20% of the Medicare-approved amount** after you meet your deductible. This is called your "Copayment."	**Out-of-pocket costs vary**—plans may have different out-of-pocket costs for certain services.

Original Medicare	Medicare Advantage (Part C)
You pay a **premium (monthly payment) for Part B**. If you choose to join a Medicare drug plan, you'll pay a separate premium for your Medicare Drug Coverage (**Part D**).	You pay the monthly **Part B premium** and may also have to **pay the plan's premium**. Plans may have a $0 premium and may help pay all or part of your **Part B** premium. Most plans include Medicare Drug Coverage (**Part D**).
There's **no yearly limit** on what you pay out of pocket, unless you have supplemental coverage—like Medicare Supplement Insurance (**Medigap**).	Plans have a **yearly limit** on what you pay out of pocket for services Medicare **Part A** and **Part B** cover. Once you reach your plan's limit, you'll pay nothing for services **Part A** and **Part B** cover for the rest of the year.
You **can get** Medigap to help pay your remaining out-of-pocket costs (like your 20% coinsurance). Or you can use coverage from a former employer or union, or Medicaid.	You **can't buy and don't need** Medigap.

Coverage

Original Medicare	Medicare Advantage (Part C)
Original Medicare covers most medically necessary services and supplies in hospitals, doctors' offices, and other health care facilities. Original Medicare doesn't cover some benefits like eye exams, most dental care services, and routine exams.	Plans must cover all of the medically necessary services that Original Medicare covers. Most plans offer **extra benefits that Original Medicare doesn't cover**—like some routine exams and vision, hearing, and dental services.
You can join a **separate Medicare drug plan** to get Medicare Drug Coverage (**Part D**).	**Medicare Drug Coverage (Part D) is included in most plans.** In most types of Medicare Advantage Plans, you can't join a separate Medicare drug plan.

In most cases, you don't have to get a service or supply approved ahead of time for Original Medicare to cover it.	In some cases, you have to get a service or supply approved ahead of time for the plan to cover it.

Foreign travel

Original Medicare	Medicare Advantage (Part C)
Original Medicare doesn't **cover care outside the United States.** You may be able to buy a Medicare Supplement Insurance (Medigap) policy that covers emergency care outside the United States. That is not obtained through Medicare.	Plans don't **cover care outside the United States.** Some plans may offer a supplemental benefit that covers emergency and urgently needed services when traveling outside the United States.

If Medicare Advantage covers "everything," why would people want Original Medicare?

The major differences are costs and accessibility.

Some people with limited financial resources have no choice but to enroll and continue in a Medicare Advantage plan (also called "Medicare HMO"). Please confirm typical costs for where you live. That can be found on the Medicare web site. This will provide you with the necessary information about the costs for Plan A, Plan B, and Plan C. Once you know your price options, you can decide if you can afford the Original Medicare, plus the supplement, plus the prescription drug plan. The cost of Part A and Part B is often taken out from an individual's social security check each month. The cost of the supplement and of the drug benefit plan is extra.

The other major reason why many people choose the Original Medicare, and not the Medicare HMO, has to do with accessibility of physicians of their choice. Not all doctors will choose to associate with HMO or provide care for their patients. There is a published Medicare fee schedule that all physicians who participate abide by. HMO compensates their physicians in a different way. Some may be full-time employees of the HMO and will receive a yearly salary. Others will be in practice and will receive a capitation fee. That means the doctor will receive a fee each month for each patient, whether a patient receives health care or not. Full-risk capitation means that the doctor will receive money each month, even if the patient does not come to see her or her. However, the same doctor is responsible for all the costs associated with that patient, usually including referrals for diagnostic tests and procedures, referrals to consultants or specialists, and all other costs. Some plans offer doctors not such a risky compensation arrangement, but regardless, the incentive on those doctors is to provide as little care as is reasonable because he or she (or their employer) makes more money. Specialists who provide care for HMO patients must negotiate their own compensation contracts each year. Often the amount offered to a doctor is a percentage of Medicare, maybe 50% or 75%, but that is highly variable between communities and states. If the HMO cannot find any specialist to contract at that level, the HMO might have to offer more to the specialist. One can see that busy doctors with few open appointments will not want to accept a fraction of Medicare when that doctor can fill the slot with a full-paying patient. That is why an HMO patient might not be able to see the specialist of his or her choice at the hospital or center where he or she usually goes for care. There are many good doctors who work in HMOs, but possibly the doctors you are now using do not. Before you join HMO or switch to HMO, make sure you ask your doctor's office if the doctor accepts the HMO you are considering.

In the past 15 years or so, a new classification of doctors was developed. This is called "concierge medicine." It is also called "retainer medicine," "membership-medicine," and "direct care." Usually, a primary care doctor will make that choice, but some specialists do as well. For a fee paid each year in January, the concierge primary care doctor agrees to limit the number of patients they care for. Often that number is around 600. A typical primary care doctor might usually follow 2,000 patients in his or her private practice. The doctor who offers concierge service promises to limit the number of patients they see each day, to spend as much time as necessary with each patient (at least 30 minutes), to call back the patient promptly (some even give out their mobile phone number), to call in all prescription refills promptly, to send out medical records to other doctor promptly when requested, and to be totally available for each patient. For doing all that, a concierge doctor might charge from $2,000 up to $7,500 per year, which can be paid monthly, although that fee may increase in the near future. In addition to that yearly fee, the doctor will continue to bill insurance (including Medicare) for any care provided or tests performed. This concept started in the wealthy communities around the United States but has now spread into other communities. One of the major complaints about doctors is the difficulty in getting in to see a doctor. That situation should never occur with a concierge doctor.

Some concierge doctors are part of a larger group network that may offer some benefits to the patients as well.

The last type of doctor is one who does not accept any insurance for payment. The patient will be told upfront that the doctor does not participate in Medicare, and the patient is expected to pay at the time of service. This type of service is not very popular but does occur often in some teaching hospitals (those associated with a medical school), but certainly not all. If you want to see such a physician, you will be told that information at the time you schedule your visit.

Once you get past the insurance/payment issues, what should you expect from your doctor and what should your doctor expect from you? First, you should expect to be seen by a doctor in a reasonable time, especially if you are acutely ill or have just received a diagnosis of a serious illness from another doctor. Access to health care has become a serious problem. At one time, less than 20 years ago, 80% of all physicians worked in 1- to 3-person groups. For a variety of reasons, fewer small group practices still exist, and they are often composed of doctors who have been together for a long time, many of whom are approaching their own retirement. Now over 70% of doctors are employed by someone else or work for a hospital or medical center, an HMO, an insurance company, a large group practice, the VA system, or even for a private equity company that has acquired physician practices and merged them together. The jargon "conveyor belt medicine" refers to those practices in which doctors are urged to see patients who need procedures that can only be done by them and leave lower-paying visits (like routine follow-ups for surgery) in the hands of a lower-paying doctor or physician extender. Yes, that is sadly true.

In addition, just trying to reach the doctor for an appointment is challenging. Rather than the phone ringing in the office of the doctor you are trying to see, often the phone is answered at a call center by a service staff who keeps the schedule of a great many doctors and has no idea of how to triage a new patient, but just follows orders in scheduling. Sounds terrible, but this happens more and more as costs of running a medical office keep rising and reimbursements from Medicare or private insurance does not keep up with inflation.

Second, your doctor should listen to you and talk to you. After all, you are paying her or him for just that. Be prepared, however, that in the days of the electronic health record (EHR) some doctors don't look at their patients eye-to-eye but look at the computer screen to document information. The major complaint against doctors is that they don't run on time. This is purely a function of how the doctor runs his or her life. There is no excuse for running an hour or 2 hours late. Yet, you may have no choice but to accept that if you like your doctor.

Third, always prepare a list of questions you have before you see your doctor each time. When you get into the examination room, you may often end up feeling angry for waiting so long that you focus your energy on complaining rather than telling the doctor what has been going on in your life.

Fourth, treat your doctor with respect. The doctor has spent an exceptionally long time in training and needs to keep up constantly with new developments in the field. By showing that respect, your doctor will treat you that way in return.

Finally, be reasonable with your expectations. A common issue is the prescribing of medications. Don't tell the doctor you want to take one of the new medications you saw on a TV commercial. Let the doctor come to you with recommendations. Also, do not put pressure on a doctor to prescribe medications that you might not really need. The most common example is the use of antibiotics for a common cold. Let the doctor decide if you have a bacterial infection (which you usually do not), for which antibiotics do nothing. There has been a tremendous increase in antibiotic resistance, contributed to by overuse of antibiotics, not to even mention what it does to your microbiome (see Chapter 7).

Last, a brief comment about the "annual physical," which has always been a part of patient's lives. There are many studies that show healthy people do not need annual physicals and that annual physicals usually don't make you healthier. Tests like blood and urine tests or EKGs without any good reason will not help you stay well and live longer. They do not help you avoid hospital stays or keep you from dying of cancer or heart disease. On the other hand, certain screening tests are indicated, like regular mammograms for women and prostate exams for men, along with periodic screening tests for colon cancer. If there are certain diseases that run in your family, you certainly need to be aware of the importance of monitoring yourself for the development of those.

Here are some reasons why you might need to see a doctor:

- You are sick.
- You have a symptom that could mean illness.
- You need to manage chronic or ongoing conditions.
- You need to check on the effects of a new medication.
- You need help with risk factor reduction like smoking or obesity.

- Prenatal care for a pregnant woman.
- Treating lifestyle issues, like family planning, sexual transmitted disease prevention, and healthy eating.
- Any other reason, based on your individual needs.

Preventive care is particularly important, although, unfortunately, it is not taught to doctors in medical school, not taught to students in school, and not practiced by most people in the country.

We feel that having a doctor available when you need them is important to us when we age. When a symptom, skin spot, or a lump do not go away, seeing a health care provider is the right thing to do.

CHAPTER 10

Traditional and Complementary Medicine

In the world of health care, there are terms that specifically need to be explained. These include the terms "complementary," "alternative," "integrative," "functional," and "progressive" health (or medicine). In general, these types of health care are used "instead of" or "in addition to" "allopathic medicine." Allopathic medicine is an archaic label for the science-based practice of conventional Western medicine, incorporating physicians, nurses, pharmacists, and therapists work together to help a person feel better. According to a report published by the National Center for Complementary and Integrative Health (NCCIH) in 2012, 38% of adults and about 12% of children use health care approaches that are not typically part of conventional medical care or that may have origins outside of Western practice. Western medicine is sometimes referred to as "allopathic" medicine.

Since so many of you may be part of the 38% or more who use some form of nonconventional health care, and because Brian is one of the leaders in the world in this field, we thought we should provide you with information, and, again, make suggestions for you to consider.

If a non-mainstream approach is used along with conventional medicine, it is considered "complementary." If a non-mainstream approach is used in place of conventional medicine, it is considered "alternative." "Integrative health" brings conventional and complementary approaches together in a coordinated way. Integrative health also emphasizes multimodal interventions, which are two or more interventions such as conventional health care approaches (*e.g.*, medication, physical therapy, rehabilitation, and psychotherapy) and complementary health approaches (*e.g.*, acupuncture, yoga, and probiotics) in various combinations, with an emphasis on treating the whole person rather than one specific organ system.

In a report from Johns Hopkins School of Medicine (Johns Hopkins Medicine, 2021), traditional alternative medicine included **homeopathic and**

Oriental practices that have been in place for centuries worldwide. They are as follows:

- Acupuncture
- Ayurveda
- Homeopathy
- Naturopathy
- Chinese or Oriental medicine

Bodywork or Touch have been used since the early days of medical care. Healing by touch is based on the idea that illness or injury in one area of the body can affect all parts of the body. With manual manipulation, the other parts can be brought back to optimum health, and the body can fully focus on healing at the site of illness. These techniques include:

- Chiropractic and Osteopathic medicine
- Massage
- Body movement therapy
- Tai Chi
- Yoga
- Sauna
- Steam
- Cold plunge
- Whirlpool

Diet and herbs are a totally different category. Over thousands of years, man has evolved from consuming a simple diet consisting of nuts, seeds, fruits, vegetables, and grains, and in some cases meat and dairy, to a diet that often consists of foods rich in fats, oils, and complex carbohydrates. (This concept has already been discussed in Chapter 1.) Nutritional excess and deficiency have become problems in today's society, leading to certain chronic diseases. According to the World Health Organization, an estimated 80% of people around the world use herbal medicine. Some people feel that allergies, premenstrual symptoms, and chronic fatigue can be treated with diet and herbs. Many dietary and herbal approaches attempt to balance the body's nutritional well-being. They may include:

- Dietary supplements
- Herbal medicines
- Nutrition or diet

External energy treatments have been practiced by some. The followers of these entities believe that external energies from objects or other sources directly affect a person's health. These treatments include:

- Electromagnetic therapy (also known as "Magnetic Field Therapy")
- Reiki
- Qigong

Mind work. Even standard or conventional medicine recognizes the power of the connection between the mind and the body. Studies have found that people actually feel better if they have good emotional and mental health. These types of therapy include:

- Meditation
- Biofeedback
- Hypnosis
- Positive psychology

Stimulation of senses. Some people believe that the senses of touch, sight, hearing, smell, and taste can have an impact on overall health and well-being. These therapies include:

- Art, dance, and music
- Visualization and guided imagery

Now, we need to talk about a very controversial topic, but one that needs to be discussed. Is there really any benefit to taking vitamins, minerals, or supplements? Facts suggest that over 70% of people over the age 65 take a multivitamin or another vitamin or mineral supplement regularly. The total price tag exceeds $12 billion per year. A study done at Johns Hopkins University (Gualiare et al., 2013) looked at a cohort of 450,000 people and concluded that multivitamins did not reduce the risk for heart disease or cancer. Another study (Cockle et al., 2000) tracked the mental functioning and multivitamin use of 5,947 men for 12 years and concluded that multivitamins did not reduce the risk for mental declines. Last, a study of 1,708 heart attack survivors (Desai et al., 2014) who took a high-dose multivitamin or placebo for up to 55 months showed that the same numbers of recurrent heart attacks, heart surgery, and death occurred in both groups.

These alternative/complementary medicines and procedures are quite common. In addition to acknowledging that over 30% of adults and 12% of children use some, or many, of these approaches, the amount of money they spend on these modalities is quite large. According to an article in the *New York Times* in 2016, which reviewed the data from the National Health and Nutrition Examination Survey (NHANES), $30.2 billion a year is spent on this type of health care. Almost half the money ($14.7 billion) was spent on visiting practitioners, like acupuncturists, homeopaths, naturopaths, chelation specialists, mind–body experts, energy-healing specialists, hypnotists, massage therapists, and traditional healers.

Natural product supplements (excluding vitamin and mineral diet supplements) in the United States alone cost $12.8 billion, and $2.7 billion was paid for self-care, including expenses for books and educational materials on diet-based therapies, guided imagery, meditation, Tai Chi, movement therapies, biofeedback, and other treatments. If you look at these facts in a different way, the $30.2 billion is not much money (only 1.1% of the nation's total health care expenditure of $2.82 trillion). The $12.8 billion spent on natural product supplements is actually 24% of the entire $54 billion spent out of pocket on prescription drugs, and the $14.7 billion in visits to alternative practitioners is almost a third of the out-of-pocket expenditures for visits to conventional physicians (Phutrakool & Pongpirul, 2022).

In the rest of the world, these so-called complementary or alternative treatments may be used by at least 50% of the population, especially those who have limited or no access to Western medicine.

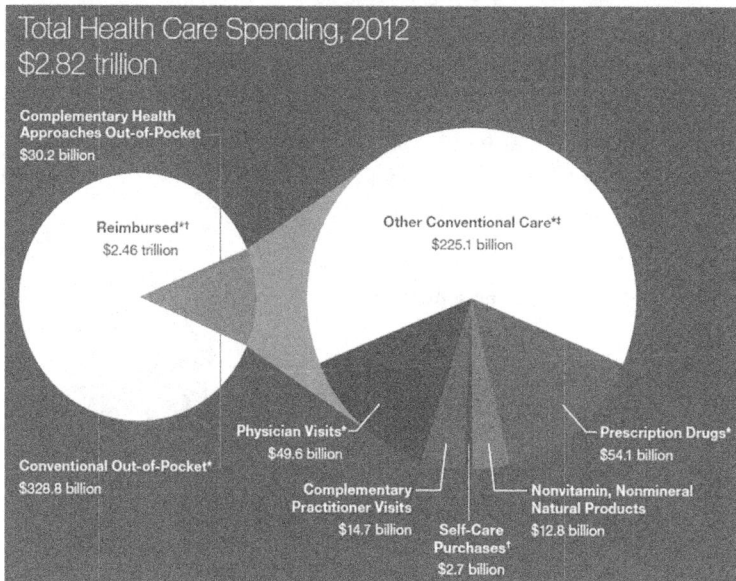

Total Health Care Spending, 2012
$2.82 trillion

Complementary Health Approaches Out-of-Pocket
$30.2 billion

Reimbursed*† $2.46 trillion

Other Conventional Care*† $225.1 billion

Physician Visits* $49.6 billion

Conventional Out-of-Pocket* $328.8 billion

Complementary Practitioner Visits $14.7 billion

Self-Care Purchases† $2.7 billion

Prescription Drugs* $54.1 billion

Nonvitamin, Nonmineral Natural Products $12.8 billion

A more recent estimation of the alternative medicine industry revenue is shown in the graph below, published by Matej Mikulic (October 2021).

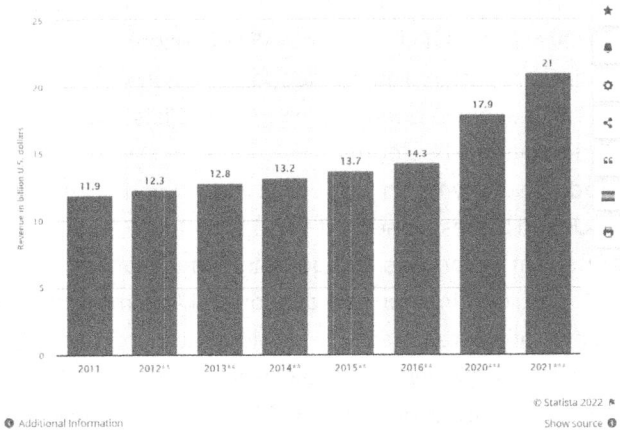

Additional information about the U.S. Dietary Supplement market can be found at https://www.grandviewresearch.com/industry-analysis/dietary-supplements-market.

The global dietary supplement market size was valued at $151.9 billion in 2021 and is expected to expand at a compounded annual growth rate of 8.9% to 2030. Increasing consumer awareness toward personal health and well-being is expected to be a key driving factor for dietary supplements and changing lifestyles. In addition, many people turn to supplements to fulfill the nutrient requirement owing to their convenience. In other words, people are more likely to take a pill or capsule than to eat healthy foods. Our society has long preached, if you are not going to eat healthy foods, just take one (or more) of our pills which will supply you with everything that you need. There are no facts to support that.

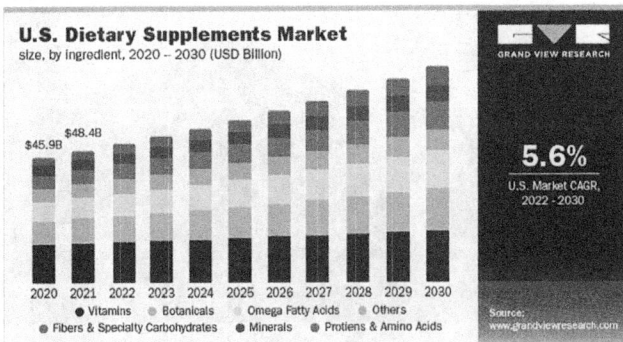

The United States has emerged as a leading market for dietary supplements in the North American region, owing to the higher spending capacity of the consumers, increasing spending on health care products, especially in the rising geriatric population such as the Baby Boomers, like all of us. Many of us, as we age, are finally showing interest in preventive health care, and there is growing interest among Baby Boomers in attaining wellness through diet and, maybe, exercise. It is the Baby Boomer population that may fuel the growing market for food supplements.

Many of us Boomers are interested in weight management, as well as dietary supplements to promote general health; bone and joint health; cardiac health; gastrointestinal health; anticancer protection; immunity boost; treatment for diabetes—controlling blood sugar levels, or even achieving the reversal of diabetes; lung diseases, and other aging- or lifestyle-related ailments. Dietary supplements might be used to fulfill nutritional deficiencies in us. As more information is obtained by scientists, there may be a demand for dietary supplements including protein and amino acids, minerals, vitamins, and omega fatty acids as new supplements to take.

In addition, increasing awareness regarding gut health owing to the increasing prevalence of irritable bowel syndrome, constipation, acid reflux, and indigestion as well as new scientific information about the importance of the microbiome in health and wellness may contribute to more of us wanting to have more information of what to take to alleviate those gastrointestinal issues. The outbreak of the COVID-19 in the year 2020 has increased the demand for immunity booster products all over the globe. Immunity-boosting vitamins, minerals, and herbs witnessed a surge in demand in 2020 which is expected to continue.

In another report published in 2022 by the Supplemental Industry (https://gitnux.org/u-s-dietary-supplement-industry-statistics/), the authors concluded that:

1. 77% of American adults consume dietary supplements. (*USA Today*)
2. Dietary supplement industry statistics reveal that 78% of the U.S. population who are 55 years old and older consume dietary supplements. (NIH)
3. Dietary supplement industry statistics show that vitamins and minerals are the most popular nutritional supplements in the United States, where 98% of supplement users are taking vitamins and minerals.
4. The value of global food supplement market in 2018 was $124.8 billion.

The real question we should all be asking is, "Are there any studies that indicate whether the use of the complementary or supplementary practices described earlier in this chapter actually work?" Many major cancer centers (like Memorial Sloan Kettering Cancer Center and M.D. Anderson Cancer Center) have entire departments of complementary medicine, which means to us, do everything that your health care provider recommends for treatment of your medical condition, but doing all the other things we mentioned earlier in this chapter might contribute to your being able to deal with your illness.

Until the answers are in, we strongly recommend listening to your health care provider if you develop a medical issue, but never replace conventional treatments (if there are any) with alternative treatments unless there are no viable options. On the other hand, adding more complementary treatments can be very beneficial. These include modifying your diet to a plant-based one, eliminating sugar from your diet (if you have cancer), and adding acupuncture, visualization, meditation, biofeedback, and body work if you have chronic pain. Always try to be aware of less conventional treatments, but always do the research yourself or in conjunction with your health care provider as to what other modalities might be available to help you.

In the area of supplements, let's take a close look at studies that are available. The passage of the Dietary Supplement Health and Education Act of 1994 opened the industry to bringing new products to market without submitting any evidence to the Food and Drug Administration (FDA) that they are safe and effective in people. This law allows products to be promoted as "supporting" the health of various parts of the body if no claim is made that they can prevent, treat, or cure any ailment. The wording appears not to stop many people from assuming that "support" means proven benefit (Brody, 2016).

Elizabeth D. Kantor *et al.* (2016), revealed that 52% of the 37,958 adults in the NHANES used one or more supplements in 2012. That number had remained stable for 12 years despite all the promotion in paid advertising and testimonials on the Internet. An editorial in the same issue of that journal, written by Dr. Pieter A. Cohen, pointed out that "supplements are essential to treat vitamin and mineral deficiencies" and that certain combinations of nutrients can help some medical conditions, like age-related macular degeneration. He added that "for the majority of adults, supplements provide little, if any, benefit." Yet despite those observations, the use of supplements and other products continues to stay stable or even grow. It has been shown that the use of a product called glucosamine–chondroitin sulfate could not relieve arthritic pain, according to the negative results of a published clinical trial in 2006 (*J Pain Palliat Care Pharmacother* 2008;22(1):39-43.)

More data from the NHANES study revealed the many reasons for the survey participants to use supplements: 45% said they took them to "improve" and 33% to "maintain" overall health; 36% of women took calcium for bone health, and 18% of men took supplements for heart health or to lower cholesterol, and only 23% used supplements because a health care provider suggested that they do so. Those supplement users were among the healthiest members of the population. They were more likely than nonusers to report being in very good or excellent health, to use alcohol moderately, to refrain from cigarette smoking, to exercise frequently, and to have health insurance. Other studies have shown that supplement use is also more frequent among those who are older, who weigh less, and who have higher levels of education and socioeconomic status. Those observations make it very hard to try to determine possible health benefits of a supplement, since a clinical study would have to control for all of those variables.

With all those equivocal or anecdotal observations, the U.S. Preventive Services Task Force, an independent group of physicians, opted not to recommend the regular use of any multivitamins to prevent cardiovascular disease or cancer in people who were not nutrient-deficient.

Now you should be asking yourself—"why do many people opt to take one or more dietary supplements?" Most people will respond with something like "nutritional insurance," knowing that they often eat erratically or fail to consume the recommended amounts of nutrient-rich vegetables and fruits. However, true nutrition specialists point out that no pill can supply all the nutrients found in wholesome foods, and many of these supplements do not even contain what they claim they do. With all that in mind, the choice of what you should take, how much you should take, where you should obtain the supplements, and even how long you should remain on the supplements are purely personal decisions. Because so many people do believe in those supplements, we felt that providing you with proper information would be a welcome opportunity to make good choices in the area of dietary supplements.

Dr. Clement has a huge wealth of knowledge in this area. Let's see what he recommends.

Which minerals, supplements, cofactors, and trace vitamins should be taken and why?

Globally soils have been so depleted from over-farming and excess chemical use that there are fewer nutrients left in the soil with the same number of plants growing on it. In 1987, leading scientists revealed that there were 90 of the 120 essential minerals missing in the soil samples taken from farms in Europe, South America, North America, and Asia. For this reason, unprocessed plant-based supplements are required to maintain biological health and energy excellence. Crucial nutrients that should be in everyone's daily menu are living forms of B_{12} which is a soil-based microorganism. We estimate that 70% of the population may lack that vitamin. When absent, it can cause neurodegenerative problems, including dementia. Another nutrient family that is often absent is Omega Oleic Acid oil. The best sources for this come from sea plants and seeds. This provides physical and mental energy and feeds the brain so that mental clarity, focus, and attunement prevail. Vitamin D, which we now know is really a hormone, has become increasingly more important since Vitamin D deficiency is associated with weak bones, impaired immune function, and predisposes one to cancer.

Minerals are equally essential and almost completely missing from farms employing commercial farming techniques. Two powerful minerals that have been lacking in our soil for a century or more are iodine and selenium. Deficiency of those minerals may alter thyroid gland function, as well as cause changes in mental health. Calcium, although rarely deficient, is important for teeth and bones, and it also assists healthy bacteria in our microbiome to resist the potential for the colon to create cancer. Magnesium is imperative since it relaxes muscles and also bonds with calcium to strengthen tissue. Iron is also important to create sufficient red blood cells. Every mineral should be considered as essential. In the case of minerals, the only type that should be considered for consumption is of the ionic (electrically charged) variety. When consuming plants in large amounts, all the minerals provided are in that form.

Biological and nutritional science now realizes that there is a symbiotic relationship between all nutrients. The disproven idea—that taking isolated types manufactured in a laboratory attempting to mimic what is believed to be found in plants—does not work. What will work instead is consuming whole plant-based foods and supplements made from them without heating them and killing the nutrient factors inherently rich with a wide variety of supporting cofactors.

Is there a guide to follow to know which supplements and how much of each we should take?

The answer to that question is not so simple. We would like everyone to take a bacterial form of B12 and a food-based variety of Vitamin D and a wide spectrum of essential minerals. Until we have available a well-studied and community-normed blood test, saliva test, or urine test, it is impossible to legitimately suggest the exact amount each person should take. It is accepted among scientists that the U.S. government standards are, at best, inadequate, and, at worse, incorrect. Dr. Colin Campbell, a biochemist and nutritionist, and Professor Emeritus at Cornell University, was involved in those studies. He commented that those government standards were "a shallow attempt, giving fleeting guidance."

It is reasonable that when one is ill, they should require higher amounts of specific nutrients. However, that is not proved. Before modern medicine's "pharmaceutical revolution," doctors had limited resources for treating people and often turned to alterations of diet to treat certain illnesses.

How does an individual know which brand to buy?

It is clear to me that over 90% of the supplements on the shelves of drug stores, grocery stores, health-food stores, vitamin stores, and even on-line stores, are cheap, ineffective knockoffs that are manmade in laboratories. Because of how these products are manufactured in laboratories, there actually may be no benefit to the body in taking them. In addition, the body's immune system may have to work harder to rid the body of those supplements. The for-profit side of this industry does not allow adequate double-blind research studies to support or refute those products, so the consumer really has no way of knowing which products to buy and to use.

Are there are tests that can be run to determine what is needed and is there a follow-up test to see if it works?

There is a company named "SpectraCell" which claims to be able to measure intracellular concentrations of so-called micro-nutrients. LetsGetChecked also claims to be able to measure levels of magnesium, copper, selenium, zinc, Vitamin D, Vitamin B12, and Vitamin E. There are probably other companies that offer similar analyses. It is not known whether the results from these analyses are accurate in diagnosing any deficiencies that correlate with clinical illness. This is an area of ongoing research that has the potential to be of great importance for health care providers.

Can we measure any outcomes from taking all those?

There are several ways to measure outcomes. The first is just plain appearance. People who are healthy actually "look healthy." They are said to have shining hair, eyes, and skin. When people are sick, they often look "sickly" whether that is caused by an illness, disease, or even nutritional deficiency. Until we know the facts about these minerals and nutrients, we all just have to practice what we think is comfortable and right. This is certainly a potentially important aspect of health, but we have no more specific recommendations to offer.

How and When to Retire

Retirement is a scary time in one's life. Many people are afraid to retire for two reasons: fear of not knowing what to do with their time and whether they will have enough money to live on. Those two issues can be extremely stress-provoking to some people. In addition, some people enter retirement with the expectation of having so much time to do some many things, yet nothing materializes, and they can become miserable.

People retire for a variety of reasons. In some cases, there is a mandatory age for retirement in the company where the individual works. Some people are so stressed and overwhelmed with working such long hours and not being able to cut back because work has always been in their lives. Other people retire for health reasons or health reasons related to their spouse. Some retire to travel and do things they never were able to do because they neither had the time nor the money to do so while working. Others are just bone-tired at the end of the workday that they come home and fall asleep on the sofa right after dinner. Retirement should be a gradual process unless an unexpected life challenge appears. Most importantly for Baby Boomers, retirement should be planned, no different than one plans a new business, a date night, or a surprise birthday party for a friend. Yet few of us ever do that. Here are some suggestions to consider.

Retire on your terms if you can. Make sure you think about what you will do after you retire. Do you want to start a new career or a new business? Do you want to travel the world with your spouse or partner while you are still physically able and have enough money to do so? Would you like to live on one cruise after another for two or three years straight? Would you like to volunteer at a school, a hospital, a nonprofit organization, or work at a ski lift punching lift tickets in exchange for your own lift ticket for the winter season? Every reason can be true.

It is our opinion that you should have three goals in mind when you make the decision to retire (Levy & Spiro, 2022):

- Do something that you are good at.
- Do something you enjoy doing.
- Do something that helps other people.

Some people will need to supplement their savings with income to make sure they do not run out of money, especially if inflation starts to get out of hand, or the stock and bond markets precipitously fall. It may be difficult to find that type of job or volunteer position, so plan for that. Otherwise, you may find yourself sitting around the swimming pool at your Florida or Arizona condominium and talk about everyone in the neighborhood, or, worse, stay at home all day, bothering your spouse to go places or do things, when your spouse is still working or already has a full day planned out.

Another major factor about retirement is to be wise about managing the money you do have and to have it invested properly and consistent with your needs. Remember, since you are no longer working, you will have no steady source of income. Where should you start to figure that out?

We recommend that you first determine how much money you spend each year. That is easier than you think. Give yourself a few hours of uninterrupted time. Open your check book(s) and add up all the checks that you wrote during the past year. Include things like mortgage payments or monthly condominium fees that are also debited automatically from your account. Add to that amount, how many personal expenses you charge to your business or expense account that will not be there when you retire. Figure out if you want to contribute money to religious or other nonprofit organizations that you support but have not funded. Think about if you want to help support your children, your grandchildren, or even your aging parents, if you are so blessed. Do those calculations for three years in a row, average them, and you should have an approximation of how much you spend each year. People may tell you that you will spend less in retirement than while you work, but Baby Boomers usually do not believe that. Most of us want to spend as much, or even more, during retirement, as we have more time to do so. Let us say, for the sake of discussion, that you need to have income to live on of approximately $100,000 per year after taxes.

Next look at what is in your retirement account or your 401K account or the equivalent. Divide that number by $100,000, and you will see if you will have enough money to live on for the number of years you plan to live with no more money coming in from investments (so-called passive income). But no one knows how long you will live and if you might run into unexpected and non-budgeted expenses like medical bills or home repairs. Most likely, you will not have enough money in that account to live on for a long time, even if you combine accounts with your spouse. Also, most retirement accounts are not in cash, and it may be an awkward time to withdraw funds from your retirement, like when the stock market has taken a significant fall in value. If you do not understand all these concepts, there are many certified financial planners available to help you, although for a fee. You probably will need to have accumulated savings to live on in addition to what you have in your retirement accounts.

That is why retirement funding should be planned, not just allowed to happen, preferably starting when you are five to ten years away from retiring. First, you should anticipate that the cost of living will be much more than it is now in five to ten years. There is no way to know what inflation will do to your savings or to the cost of living. A good rule of thumb is to double the amount of money you are spending now to need for your retirement. It is always better to have more than enough money to live on in retirement, than not enough. During those preretirement years (more than five years before you anticipate realistically retiring), start investing any surplus funds (*i.e.*, money that you do not spend every year) in growth-type investments. For most people, growth investments are usually in the stock market, although limited partnerships and private investments may be an option for some who understand how those types of investments work. The problem with having everything you own in stocks (also called "equities") is that there could be a sharp decline in the value of your stocks (called a "correction"), and that fall could last many years before it recovers. That is why when you approach and then reach retirement time, you might want to have a very low percentage of your entire investment portfolio in equities. What if you planned to use the $500,000 you had accumulated in your retirement account for the funds you would be living on during retirement, only to have a massive "correction" six months before you plan to retire, and that $500,000 is now only $300,000.) Once you stop working, there is no way to replace invested assets at that point unless you go back to work, which might be an impossible task. Unfortunately, you may have no choice if you cannot cut back on your spending to make up that deficit.

Therefore, we advise making a slow change in your investment portfolio starting about ten years before you plan to retire. Rather than keeping nearly all of your investments in the stock market, regardless of how well the stock market has treated you over the past few years, you might start looking at income-producing investments. There are a number of such options for you to consider, all of which have different projected rates of return and different risks associated. It is always a good idea to diversify your investments in many different types of income-producing investments, as you never know which one sector will be the most successful. Those income-generating investments include:

- Cash (money market)
- Certificates of deposit (CDs)
- Dividend-producing stocks, preferred stocks
- ETFs (Exchange Traded Funds) that invest in income-producing stocks
- Corporate bonds, taxable municipal bonds, tax-free municipal bonds, or bond funds
- Annuities
- Limited partnerships
- Personal loans, first mortgages, second mortgages, bridge loans
- Real estate, wholly owned
- Real estate partnerships
- Real Estate Investment Trusts (REITs)
- Royalties
- Another business

It might be prudent to start the transition from owning equities to owning income-producing investments around ten years before your planned retirement. In retirement, it is not a good idea to invest in speculative-type investments or even in the stock market, unless you feel sure that your investment portfolio–generated funds are way more than you will need in retirement. In other words, do your investments provide enough passive income to live on? Still another way to t about these types of investments is that they are investments that earn money for you while you sleep.

You should never invest in anything you do not understand, or give money to people you do not know, no matter how great an investment may be pitched to you. You might seek the services of a financial planner or a wealth manager, but please learn enough to make sure you know what to tell such an adviser about your needs and your risk tolerances, the timeframe you are facing, and your past experiences in the world of investing. If you do choose a money manager or a wealth manager, make sure you and your manager both agree on a benchmark (like the Dow-Jones Investment

Average or the S&P 500 Average) to judge how well the manager is doing compared to what you could have done with passive investing (buying only Index Funds). Knowing how to evaluate their performance is important. That is beyond the scope of this book.

Do I need to have a will, power of attorney, and living will?
Yes, you do. You should find an attorney who specializes in preparing these types of documents and meet with that person to document your wishes.

Do I have to distribute my assets equally to my children or grandchildren?
No, this is purely your choice. There is nothing in writing to demand that. Talk things over with the estate attorney that you choose.

The world of investing is too complicated for me. Can I keep everything I own in bonds?
Certainly, some people do that. But remember, every investment is associated with some type of risk. Stocks can fall in value. Companies can withhold distributing dividends. In the case of bonds, you are locked into a return calculated when you buy the bond. Even if the value of the bond on the open market changes from day to day, you will still collect the same amount of income each year. If there is rampant inflation, the buying power of your income will drop. That is why we recommend diversification of your income-producing investments, in case one sector outperforms the others in any given year.

My spouse runs all the family investments, including making all the investment decisions, writing all the checks, and even preparing all the documents needed for my CPA to prepare our joint tax return. What will happen if he or she dies first?
This is always an issue for middle- or high-net-worth couples, especially if one or both are professionals. There is almost always one person who runs the family business and just looks to the other spouse for blessings, not for decisions. This issue should be talked about together and with your estate attorney. Sometimes there is a child who can take over the financial management, but sometimes there is a need for a commercial trustee like an officer of a bank or trust company, who takes over those roles. Do not wait to the last minute to find such a person. Start interviewing those advisers while you can and try to find a person whom you can relate to and who will follow your expressed investment goals and objectives. For example, if you believe

in income-producing real estate to provide income to live on during retirement, but the trust officer only knows about stocks, the first thing that might happen is that the real estate gets sold, solely because the officer does not understand that investment. That may not be part of your objectives.

What does the term "Required Minimum Distribution" (RMD) mean, and how does that apply to me?

According to the AARP (American Association of Retired Persons), Required Minimum Distributions (RMDs) generally are minimum amounts that a retirement plan account owner must withdraw annually starting with the year that he or she reaches 72 years of age (70 ½ if you reach that age before January 1, 2020), and if later, the year in which he or she retires. Your withdrawals will be included in your taxable income except for any part that was taxed before (your basis) or that can be received tax-free (such as qualified distributions from designated Roth accounts). This means that you will have to withdraw a specific amount of money from your retirement plan, and you will be taxed on those funds. There are specific ways you can withdraw those funds that may have tax advantages. Please consult your accountant or tax adviser. Those requirements may be changed by our government from time to time, so make sure you or your financial adviser follows this area closely.

As you are reading this chapter, you might have asked yourself, why is this information included in a book about longevity? We feel that living a long life only to have to deal with financial issues can be very stressful in your older years. Even worse would be to outlive your finances and need to rely on your children, if you have any. Plus, there is a real concern that social security might not be there sometime in the future without radical changes in its own financial structure. Moreover, social security, by itself, may not provide enough money for an individual to live on unless that person has significant savings outside of social security, like a retirement plan, 401K plan, or personal savings. Last, when you are much older, you might not have the mental skills to manage the money you need to live on. For those reasons, we wanted to provide a brief overview of what you might consider doing now or in the near future.

CHAPTER
12 Inflammation

An area of active investigation is the relationship between aging and inflammation. All of you have experienced or seen inflammation. If you burn yourself with a match, touch poison ivy in a park, cut your finger peeling potatoes, or even twist your ankle while playing tennis, you have experienced inflammation. Pain, swelling, warmth, and redness are the hallmark signs of inflammation. That is one type of inflammation. This type is the body's way to fight infection and heal damage. It is called "acute inflammation."

Acute inflammation is the body's response to an injury, illness, or infection. There is a cascade of events that occur, starting with white blood cells congregating in the area. This process is designed to heal the injury or the infection. Depending upon the type of injury or infection, this inflammatory response will slowly resolve over hours to days.

There is another type of inflammation that is called "chronic inflammation." Although this type of inflammatory reaction is not often discussed, many scientists feel that chronic inflammation may be the most important factor in the development of chronic illnesses and aging. This chronic inflammation is characterized by unresolved and uncontrolled inflammation with multivariable low-grade, chronic, and systemic responses that exacerbate the aging process and age-related chronic diseases (Chung *et al.*, 2019).

One type of chronic inflammation is the development of autoimmune diseases. Those conditions include rheumatoid arthritis (not osteoarthritis. which is very common), insulin-dependent (type 1) diabetes mellitus, regional enteritis, ulcerative colitis, Graves' disease (overactive thyroid), Hashimoto's disease (underactive thyroid), systemic lupus erythematosus, alopecia areata (an unusual type of hair loss), some types of vasculitis (inflammation of blood vessels), psoriasis, myasthenia gravis, scleroderma, and multiple sclerosis. Those diseases are all associated with an inflammatory response in one or more organs of the body, often ending up with scarring or fibrosis and eventual altered or loss of function of that organ. The NIH (National Institutes of Health) estimates that autoimmune diseases affect between 5% and 8% of the U.S. population. It is thought that these diseases are caused by the body producing antibodies directed against an organ. Even though most antibodies are useful and protective (fighting off infection, cancer surveillance, and fighting bacteria), antibodies produced by patients with autoimmune diseases are usually harmful or destructive. These types of conditions are common and tend to run in families.

There is another form of chronic inflammation that is common in seniors. Some of the vague, nonspecific symptoms of chronic inflammation include feeling tired all the time, gaining weight, headaches, rashes that come and go, unexplained muscle and joint aches, and even gastrointestinal symptoms like constipation or diarrhea. Most people refer to those symptoms as symptoms of "getting old," but they may be symptoms of chronic inflammation.

Researchers working in the field of longevity are trying to understand aging and have proposed a role for chronic inflammation as a part of the process of aging and age-related diseases. This is consistent with the concept that aging is a disease, not an inevitable loss of organ function associated with growing old. It is thought that aging results from an interaction of genetic, environmental, and epigenetic factors (Sanada *et al.*, 2018). (Epigenetic factors are factors that allow cells to control gene activity without changing the DNA sequence.) Chronic inflammation is thought to be a risk factor in many age-related diseases. These include atherosclerosis, diabetes, and cancer, along with physical disability and cognitive decline (Freund *et al.*, 2010).

Several factors have been proposed that can initiate and perpetuate chronic inflammation. These include aging itself, eating an unhealthy diet, a decline in amount of sex hormones, and smoking. It has been noted that aged individuals have consistently elevated levels of cytokines (cell signaling molecules that aid cell-to-cell communication in immune responses). Two of these cytokines are interleukin-6 (IL-6) and tumor necrosis factor-α (TNF-α) which may induce muscle atrophy and cancer through DNA damage (Singh & Newman, 2011). It is thought that excess fat in the organs of obese individuals can also produce both IL-6 and TNF-α. Cigarette smoke contains multiple producers of inflammation, and chronic smoking increases the production of IL-6 and TNF-α, as well as another cytokine, interleukin-β. Still another cytokine is CRP (C-reactive protein), which is a protein produced in the liver in response to elevations of IL-6. Mental stress and even periodontal disease have been reported as causes of chronic inflammation.

Certain factors are associated with an elevation of these markers of chronic inflammation:

- Visceral fat (fat found in organs rather than the fat found under the skin) and high-fat diets.

- Sex hormones. It is known that the sex hormones (estrogen in women and testosterone in men) decline with age. Studies suggest that estrogen and testosterone inhibit the secretion of IL-6 (Pottratz & Bellido, 1994). Also, levels of IL-6 increase after the onset of menopause, suggesting the importance of estrogen in regulating IL-6.
- Smoking
- Depression
- Stress

Interestingly, long-term exercise is associated with lower levels of these markers (Nicklas *et al.*, 2008).

What are some of the consequences of chronic inflammation?

- Cardiovascular disease
  In younger patients, there are traditional risk factors for heart disease and stroke. They are hypertension, elevated levels of low-density lipoprotein (LDL) cholesterol, diabetes, smoking, secondhand smoke exposure, obesity, unhealthy diet, and lack of physical activity. The predictive value of these risk factors, however, tends to decline with age. So, in older persons IL-6 and TNF-α may be more predictive of the risk of cardiovascular disease than the factors for the disease in younger patients. Many scientific studies have shown chronic inflammation to be an integral part of the atherosclerotic process.
- Diabetes
  TNF-α seems to contribute to insulin resistance in patients with type 2 diabetes.
- Cancer
  IL-6 and CRP have been associated with different types of cancer, especially multiple myeloma and lymphatic cancers.
- Osteopenia and osteoporosis
- Chronic anemia
- Regional enteritis
- Polymyalgia rheumatica (PMR)

There are other conditions that seem to be related to chronic inflammation. They include:

- Fragility (decline in strength, unintentional weight loss, fatigue, low physical activity level, slow walking speed, and falls)

- Cognitive decline (including the dementia associated with Alzheimer's disease and vascular dementia)
- Mortality

An interesting model was proposed by Sanada *et al.* (2018) and is adapted here:

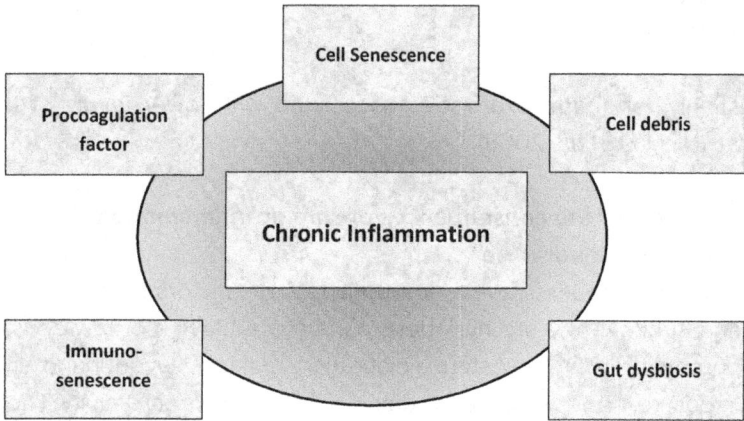

This model suggests that there may be several factors that contribute to the chronic inflammation associated with aging. This model provides a possible explanation of the pathophysiology of the aging process and gives us suggestions of what we can do now, until the scientists provide us with more specific biological treatments for delaying or reversing aging.

Many tissues in the elderly have chronic inflammation, thought to be mediated in part, by the same cytokines (IL-6, IL 1-β, TNF-α). These cytokines have been postulated to affect certain essential cascades (events that occur in the body in response to an external or internal stress) caused by insulin and erythropoietin secretion (a hormone affects the formation of red blood cells in response to low oxygen levels).

Cell Debris

Cell debris accumulation is an active area of research, with scientists looking at its cause, its removal, and even its prevention, as a way to slow down the aging process (see Chapter 13). One theory is that cell debris and immunoglobulin accumulation due to impaired removal from within the cells may be a potent trigger for the immune system activation leading to chronic inflammation. It is known that glycosylation (attaching a glucose molecule to a protein) is a common modification of a protein. Glycosylated proteins play specific roles in the interactions between cells and molecules. The sugar chains that are N-linked to the amino acid asparagine may be a new bio-marker of natural aging. This biomarker seems to be present in a rare condition called "progeria" or premature aging associated with very early death. This same or similar biomarker may be a trigger for autoimmune and inflammatory diseases. A specific part of the cell is called "mitochondria," which is the energy-producing organelle. Alterations in molecular patterns within these mitochondria may be factors in the chronic inflammation associated with aging and degenerative diseases (Zhang et al., 2010).

Gut dysbiosis

Many older people frequently complain about chronic constipation. This is likely caused by a disturbance in the microbiome, the bacteria that populate the gastrointestinal track (see Chapter 7). The gut mucosa and microbiota of elderly people tends to change with age. It is known that the gut microbiota of elderly people displays decreased diversity compared to that seen in younger people. The abundance of certain anti-inflammatory microbiota, such as Clostridium cluster XIVa, Bifidobacterium, and F. Prausnitzii are diminished in aged individuals. The levels of inflammatory cytokines are inversely correlated with levels of Bifidobacterium. Changes in the gut microbiota in aged people might increase susceptibility to infectious agents by pathologic bacteria or may even trigger chronic inflammation or even autoimmunity. In fact, different stool microbiota profiles were found in healthy "community-dwelling elderly" compared to those living in long-term care facilities (Claesson et al., 2011). It was suggested that a marked difference in food consumption might account for the differences seen and might imply a novel way to prolong health over the years.

Cell Senescence

Cell senescence (or aging) is another area of active research. This process can be defined as an irreversible cell cycle arrest driven by a variety of events. This may include telomere shortening, genotoxic stress (exposure to DNA-damaging agents and subsequent energy expenditures by a cell to repair DNA damage), mitogen stimuli (nonspecific stimulants of immune cells which lead to immune cell activation), and the production of cytokines, all of which result in the activation of p53 tumor suppressor (which causes growth arrest, DNA repair, and apoptosis—cell death). It is evident that the number of senescent cells in organs increases with age and this increase is associated with the production of inflammatory cytokines that can cause chronic low-grade inflammation. There have been animal studies showing that the progression of certain age-related conditions, like atherosclerosis and osteoarthritis, are reduced by clearing the cells in an animal model of the senescent cells (Jeon et al., 2017). This work has led to ongoing research in medications that can remove these senescent cells or reprogram the cells to improve the life span of aging people (see Chapter 13).

Immunosenescence

Immunosenescence refers to the age-related changes in the regulation of the immune system that is characterized by persistent inflammatory responses. It seems that immunosenescence increases the susceptibility of the body to autoimmune diseases, malignancy, and infections. It may even impair wound healing. It is thought that chronic inflammation can accelerate the immunosenescence process.

Coagulation and Fibrinolysis System

Increased coagulation and fibrinolysis (blood clotting) in the elderly has been implicated in enhanced inflammation (Chu, 2011). Blood coagulation is a complex cascade of events involving what are called "coagulation factors." Factors V, VII, Viii, and IX have been reported to increase in healthy humans as they age. The increased levels of coagulation factors during normal aging might account for the higher cardiovascular risk observed in the elderly. The science behind this area is beyond the content of our book. There is one theory that a specific coagulation factor Xa in atherosclerotic plaques might enhance cellular senescence (Sparkenbaugh et al., 2014).

   In acute inflammation, the inflammatory process stops after the offending agent (the burn, the plant, the cut, the ankle twist) is over. That allows the body to heal itself. Low-grade chronic inflammation tends to occur in older people, which often leads to dysfunction of organs. There is even evidence that the development of conditions like cancer, cardiovascular disease, neurodegenerative disease (like Alzheimer's), type 2 diabetes, osteoarthritis, frailty, and osteoporosis is associated with low-grade elevations of circulating inflammatory mediators. Further work needs to be done to better understand the interaction between environmental factors, lifestyle, and new (or revisited) biological products that can slow down or reverse aging at the cellular level.

What can we do right now?

We should first separate the prevention of a disease from the treatment of the disease once it appears. Most doctors know how to treat the complications of a heart attack, but few focus on the prevention of the atherosclerotic process. Most doctors know about all the medications that can be used to lower the blood sugar of a patient with type 2 diabetes, but few present the proper way to prevent the disease before it appears. Certain neurodegenerative diseases (Alzheimer's disease, Parkinson's disease), some forms of cancer, and maybe even obesity might be approached differently if we, as health care providers, focus on early diagnosis and prevention, focusing on lifestyle changes, rather than waiting until symptoms or signs appear and then resorting to medication or surgery.

If we choose to look at aging as a disease, we need to focus on the delaying of the aging process right now, especially those of us who are Baby Boomers and have reached the milestone that we might even be called "elderly" (G-d forbid).

There are two different avenues for prevention of age-related complications. One, we call "lifestyle" and the other we call "biologics." As described in length in Chapters 1-6 of this book, we feel that proper diet, intense exercise, brain stimulation, community involvement, spirituality, and maybe sex will provide a great foundation to remain with us as we age. Those are the factors included in "lifestyle."

The diet component is interesting as there are many foods that are considered anti-inflammatory. They include:

- Ripe fruits like cherries, blueberries, strawberries, tomatoes, and oranges
- Green leafy vegetables, like spinach, kale, collard greens, and, especially, all sprouts
- Sprouted nuts and seeds
- Whole grains
- Healthy oils like organic avocado oil, walnut oil, sesame oil, macadamia oil, chia oil, and olive oil

In addition, there are foods that are considered inflammatory foods that are processed and are high in sugar. Consideration should be made to eliminate them as much as we can from our diets now. They include:

- Soda
- Fried foods
- White bread, cookies, cakes
- All animal flesh (red meat, fowl, fish) and eggs

- All dairy products
- All products containing sugar, either alone or added to foods, including table sugar, honey, maple syrup, and agave

Scientists are working on anti-aging drugs that we call "Biologics." These are described in Chapter 13. They include aspirin, statins, ACE (angiotensin-converting enzyme) inhibitors (captopril, lisinopril, and others), ARB (angiotensin II receptor blockers, such as losartan), metformin, rapamycin, NAD+, and fisetin. These medications either alone, or in combination, may actually be able to increase longevity. However, long-term population studies using universally accepted biomarkers to monitor improvement still need to be done. In fact, there are many clinical trials in process attempting to study just that. Again, see Chapter 13.

We do believe that with a combination of the proper lifestyle and perhaps the use of specific anti-aging biologics (when available), it will be possible for all of us to "beat the chronic inflammation syndrome" and live to 120 years.

CHAPTER 13

For the Future

As we have said before, humans have long been looking for ways to extend their lives. From the Sumerian Epic of Gilgamesh (an epic poem from ancient Mesopotamia) to the Egyptian Edwin Smith medical papyrus (written around 1501 BC and named after Edwin Smith who bought in in 1862) to the Taoist, Ayurveda practitioners, the alchemists, and even philosophers like Francis Bacon, René Descartes, Benjamin Franklin, and Nicolas Condorcet, humans have thought about and written about ways to live longer. In the late 1800s, there was a surge in scientific optimism and therapeutic activism, including the pursuit of life extension studies. Sociologist James Hughes (Executive Director of the Institute for Ethics and Emerging Technologies and faculty member at Trinity College) claims that science has been tied to a narrative of conquering death since the Age of Enlightenment and even quotes Francis Bacon's novel, New Atlantis (published in 1626) wherein scientists worked toward delaying aging and prolonging life. Biologist Alexis Carrel (1873–1944) was inspired by a belief in indefinite human life span that he developed after experimenting with cells (Hughes, 2011).

Around the latter part of the 20th century, products were produced and sold as ways to extend one's life. There were treatments, infusions, vitamins, and supplements offered for sale. FDA got involved with regulatory and legal struggles and even seized merchandise resulting in prolonged criminal charges that were eventually dismissed (Faloon, 2002).

To that effect in 2021, the anti-aging market worldwide was $62.5 billion U.S. dollars with the prediction of over $90 billion dollars for 2027 (Statisca)... Some critics of private research dispute the portrayal that "aging is a disease." Some scientists have criticized the anti-aging industry in response to a claim that the entire aging industry shows unscrupulous profiteering from the sale of unproven anti-aging supplements (Olshansky et al., 2002). Other scientists suggest that people buy anti-aging products to obtain a "hoped-for self" (e.g., keeping a youthful skin) or to avoid a feared self (e.g., looking old). Research shows that when consumers pursue a hoped-for self, it is their expectations of success that most strongly drive their motivation

(Sobh & Martin, 2011). To that effect, in 2020, the global anti-aging market was estimated to be worth about $58.5 billion (Statista Research Department, March 18, 2022).

Even though life extension may be possible, there are no international or national programs focused on radical life extension funded by governments. It is said that some tech innovators and Silicon Valley entrepreneurs have become investors in anti-aging research. These include Jeff Bezos (Amazon), Larry Ellison (Oracle), and Peter Thiel (PayPal). They have invested in companies like Altos Labs, a company pursuing biological reprogramming, and Calico Labs, another company focusing on reprogramming. It is said that these people have a "longevity mindset." What is that? Most people take the aging process for granted. If they're disciplined, healthy, and lucky, they'll get 20 or so years of youth, start declining in their 40s, and die sometime between 60 and 80. They accept that life expectancy is 81.2 years for females and 76.4 years for males—nothing they can do, just "take the lemons and make lemonade." Who can blame them? Nearly every human institution—governments, the insurance industry, medicine, religion—is organized around this mindset.

The Anti-Longevity Mindset is "mortality is inevitable; youth is fleeting." So, the Longevity Mindset is "mortality is avoidable, youth is extendable." If that sounds shocking to you, you're not the only one. For years, scientists supporting a Longevity Mindset were shunned, and, as a result, longevity studies were tabled for fear of losing grant funding. Ultimately, *aging is a disease*—a disease that many of the most powerful people on the planet believe can be slowed, stopped, even reversed.

Many areas of research are very technical, and their results are far from clinical use just yet. These include innovations like genome sequencing, RNA transcriptomics, Wnt pathway modifiers, vaccines, CRISPR, liquid biopsies, CAR-T cells, gene therapy, exosomes, and stem cell therapy, which are just a sampling of the technologies that the world's billionaires are fast-tracking.

The rest of this chapter will deal with products you can obtain yourself, whether it be from an organization that you read about online and buy their products, a longevity center that you go to either in the United States or overseas, a health care provider who specializes in anti-aging medicine, to products you might buy in your local health-food store. We will try to present our honest opinion about whether any of these products are worth taking, including their potential side effects, and then try to cover the most likely candidates for promoting longevity. As we always say, we want to present you with information only and do not recommend that you take any of the products. We just want our readers to be aware of what is out there so that intelligent decisions can be made.

The first thing that must be questioned in deciding whether to try a new treatment is the model used to judge efficacy of that treatment. Most longevity studies are performed in budding yeast, nematode worms, fruit flies, and mice. The advantage to using those species is that they age quickly. That means a research study can be done in weeks or perhaps two months with results that can be obtained relatively quickly. Researchers can screen thousands of potential products or medications that affect the aging process of yeast, worms, and fruit flies, just by measuring the life span of that model. Mouse studies are more complicated since their life spans are three or four years. Studies on mice take much more time and are, therefore, much more expensive. In addition, mice studies are associated with many more regulations and bureaucracy. The major reason for mice studies is that scientists can actually look at tissues and organs to look at specific changes that may occur at the tissue level or even molecular level. The message is that the bigger the animal, the more tissue that is available for investigation. Dogs are other animals that are often used in anti-aging studies. They live in a similar environment as humans and often are susceptible to the same diseases that affect humans. However, dogs live longer than mice, making the studies even more difficult to perform. On the other hand, if a scientist does find changes in the tissues of dogs, those findings may be more relevant for human aging. The next species to consider are primates (apes, monkeys, chimpanzees, gorillas). A rhesus monkey can live 25 to 30 years. Marmosets are shorter lived, but those animals have not been used extensively in scientific research; therefore, observations on their longevity may not be as significant as in monkeys.

The rest of this chapter is filled with scientific studies and terms that may not be understood by the readers. Feel free to skim those parts and read the conclusions. Our intention is to present information of practical use to our readers. The takeaway section will tie everything together.

We, as clinicians at heart, are only interested in human aging, so we want to base our recommendations on results in humans. Because of the life span of the average person being around 80, it would take decades to know for sure if some type of intervention has worked, especially if the treatment was started early in life. It is hard to make recommendations on a specific product, molecule, diet, exercise program, or even social changes, without studies done on humans using appropriate controls.

We will start by discussing if there are any biomarkers of aging that scientists could use to test new interventions instead of relying only on life extension as measured in years. What is a "biomarker"? According to the National Cancer Institute (NCI), a biomarker is a biological molecule found in blood, other body fluids, or tissues that is a sign of a normal or abnormal process or a condition or a disease. A biomarker may be used to see how well the body responds to a treatment for a disease or condition. It is also called "molecular marker" or "signature molecule." An example of a biomarker might be monitoring ApoB levels to judge the effectiveness of a new cholesterol-lowering medication. In the case of longevity or biological aging, scientists would like to have something that is predictive at either the individual level or the population level of future health outcomes, mortality, and functional outcomes like disease reduction. Some people say we already have such biomarkers. Just a quick glance at someone who is morbidly obese, with severe muscle weakness, lack of exercise stamina, and known multiple medical problems versus a person who is fit, muscular, and well-toned. The fit person most likely will live longer. But that type of observation is difficult to quantitate. There has been a search for something that could be used to measure the results of intervention studies. Some biomarkers currently under investigation include: sCD12 scavenger receptor cysteine-rich type 1 protein (CD 163), CD5 molecule-like (CD5L), neural cell adhesion molecule (CD56), soluble CD40 ligand (CDL40L), chemokine (C-X-C motif) ligand 16 (CXCL16), stromal cell–derived factor 1 (CDF1), dipeptidyl-peptidase 4 (DPP4), interleukin-6 receptor beta (SGP 130), sRAGE, and myeloperoxidase (MPO). CD14 serves as a positive control in investigations of dementia (Fang, *et al.*, 2022).

A quick Google search results in many companies that market biomarkers for aging. We have not investigated any of them, but they include the following:

- TruAge Complete Collection: suite of epigenetic aging reports and aging algorithms.
- SomaScan: aptamer-based proteomics with the development of a proprietary slow off–rate modified aptamer. Aptamers are short, single-stranded DNA or RNA (ssDNA or ssRNA) molecules that can selectively bind to a specific target, including proteins, peptides, carbohydrates, small molecules, toxins, and even live cells.
- Epigenetic Testing Kit: methylation sites from which saliva samples can accurately measure biological age through an at-home epigenetic testing kit.
- SpectraCell: a blood test for micronutrients that may have some ability to estimate biological age (see Chapter 10).
- Botechne: measures many inflammatory biomarkers.

There are also many other tests commercially available. Some biomarkers reflect biological age but are not necessarily the same as a biomarker that reflects the rate of aging. Functional biomarkers would be the ideal situation. Those might include a product of some kind that can make a person's heart beat stronger, liver work more efficiently, or brain function better. If scientists could come up with something that improves the function of multiple organs, they could make a case that the intervention is modulating some underlying biology of aging. Right now, scientists are using clinical biomarkers. Matt Kaeberlein, Ph.D., Professor of Pathology at the University of Washington, has noted some of them:

- ApoB
- Cardiovascular efficiency
- Fat-free mass index
- Glucose disposal
- Inflammatory markers
- VO_2 max (the maximum rate of oxygen consumption measured during incremental exercise, that is, exercise of increasing intensity)
- Insulin signaling
- Lipid markers
- Muscle mass
- Muscle strength

Another concept discussed by researchers is "epigenetic clocks." These are chemical modifications to either the DNA or to the histones that pack the DNA by the use of chemical modifications such as methylation and acetylation. One of the difficulties with these epigenetic clocks is that a company will often pair the results of a test with the recommendations to purchase certain supplements. This may be morally dishonest, and considered profiteering, as there are no scientific studies to support any of their findings. What the results of these tests might do is to broaden the appeal of the field to the general public or to cause them to make healthier lifestyle choices, such as to improve one's diet or to begin an exercise program. But it is still a bit dishonest to claim to people that a company or a laboratory can measure biological age with any precision, despite many companies doing just that. Dr. Kaeberlein says that these same companies are often also selling a product that they claim will reverse one's biological age. "That is just snake oil." He suggested that perhaps the FDA should step in.

With all the skepticism out there about companies selling biomarkers or epigenetic marker tests, and recommending a solution in the form of a supplement, vitamin, or other product (taken orally or by intravenous infusion), there are also people who recommend more conventional tests and intervention, many of which have no scientific backing and the supplements they recommend are not even available in the United States.

If you, as a consumer, are so inclined to experiment with any of these therapies, perhaps you would be best off doing so under the supervision of a specialist in aging, such as those who work at one of the major medical institutions mentioned later in this chapter. Some of the products that have been recommended over the years, along with our comments about them, are as follows:

Human Growth Hormone (HGH)

HGH has been used since 1985 when two companies first developed a biosynthetic form. Prior to that date, growth hormone was extracted from animal pituitary glands and used on humans, sometimes with disastrous results. Human pituitary extracts were stopped many years ago after an "epidemic" of a neurological condition called "Creutzfeldt-Jakob Disease," which is a neurodegenerative disease. Once HGH was produced in the lab by pharmaceutical companies, the use of human pituitary extracts was terminated. HGH is used to treat growth hormone deficiency and, occasionally, short stature caused by certain medical conditions. The increased availability of HGH meant experimentation with other applications for the hormone in off-label uses. One such use was the explosion of black-market HGH use by athletes to improve their performance. Though "house-sized" athletes never materialized, HGH continued to be a favorite drug for doping, particularly because it was difficult to detect in tests. For a while, competitive cyclists used HGH in combination with other performance-enhancing medications to improve their racing times. That type of "doping" is now forbidden. In addition, it is known that growth hormone decreases with age, so it seemed reasonable that HGH use might prolong lives. The work with HGH and longevity was based only on animal studies. There are mixed studies to determine whether HGH therapy modulates the aging process in humans and whether the direction of its effect is positive or negative (Sattler, 2013). In fact, the American Medical Association has been critical of anti-aging hormone therapies in general (Japsen, 2009).

Piracetam

Piracetam is a chemical made in a lab. In some countries in Europe, it is used as a drug to improve memory and brain function. In the United States, some manufacturers sell piracetam as a dietary supplement. However, the U.S. Food and Drug Administration (FDA) does not consider piracetam to be a legal dietary supplement.

Piracetam has been used for breath-holding attacks, seizure disorder (epilepsy), dizziness (vertigo), dyslexia, and a movement disorder often caused by antipsychotic drugs (tardive dyskinesia). It has also been used for dementia, schizophrenia, sickle cell disease, and many other conditions, but there is no good scientific evidence to support any of these uses. Even though piracetam might have some use for a condition called "myoclonus," we could not find any studies, human or otherwise, that showed this medication increases longevity.

DHEA

Dehydroepiandrosterone (DHEA) is a hormone derived from cholesterol and pregnenolone. It is produced by the adrenal glands and in smaller amounts in the testes in males and the ovaries in females. DHEA acts as a precursor for the production of sex hormones—testosterone and estrogen. It also has direct hormonal effects of its own throughout the body.

As DHEA levels drop with age, less testosterone and estrogen are produced. Low levels of these sex hormones contribute to loss of vitality and eventual frailty in older men and women. Lower DHEA levels are tied to other health problems and a diminished quality of life. In older men, **low** testosterone results in erectile dysfunction, a drop in libido, loss of muscle mass and bone density, a tendency toward depression, and slowing brain function. In older women, low estrogen levels are associated with a loss of libido, along with hot flashes, mood swings, fatigue, headaches, thinning of the bones, and risk for bone fractures.

But does DHEA replacement or supplementation increase longevity and what are its potential side effects? DHEA and its sulfate ester (DHEA-S) are the most abundant steroids in humans. DHEA levels fall with age in men and women, reaching values sometimes as low as 10% to 20% of those encountered in young individuals. Studies point toward several potential roles of DHEA, mainly through its hormonal end-products, making this decline clinically relevant. Unfortunately, even if positive effects of DHEA on muscle, bone, cardiovascular disease, and sexual function seem rather robust, extremely few studies are large enough and/or long enough for conclusions regarding its effects on aging. Moreover, because it has been presented as a "fountain of youth" equivalent, over-the-counter preparations lacking pharmacokinetic and pharmacodynamic data are widely used worldwide.

Nevertheless, data on the safety profile of long-term DHEA supplementation are still lacking (Samaras *et al.*, 2013). Mayo Clinic says that
there are concerns that using DHEA as a supplement might increase
the risk of hormone-sensitive cancers, including prostate, breast, and
ovarian cancers. The National Collegiate Athletic Association has
banned DHEA use among athletes.

Vinpocetine

According to WebMD, Vinpocetine is a manmade chemical, similar to
a substance found in the periwinkle plant (Vinca minor). In Europe, it's
sold as a drug called "Cavinton." Vinpocetine might increase blood flow
to the brain and protect brain cells (neurons) against injury. People use
vinpocetine for memory, dementia, stroke, hearing loss, and many other
conditions, but there is no good scientific evidence to support most of
these uses. Although vinpocetine may be a cognitive enhancement
medication, we could not find any studies documenting increased longevity in animals or humans.

GH3 or KH3

GH3 (Gerovital) is the grandmother of modern anti-aging supplements. Since it was first introduced to the Western world in the early
1950s by its inventor, Rumanian gerontologist Dr. Ana Aslan, GH3 has
been the subject of both intense marketing hype and glamor, as well
as heated scientific controversy. The marketing hype has been in part
fueled by the glamor attached to GH3's many famous users. Celebrity
columnists reported regulars at Dr. Aslan's Rumanian clinic during the
1950s and 1960s, such as German Chancellor Konrad Adenauer, Win-
ston Churchill, Bob Hope, Cary Grant, Marilyn Monroe, Jack Benny,
and Prince Rainer, among other celebrities. The scientific controversy
surrounding GH3 has stemmed in part through confusion and disa-
greement regarding both the chemical identity of GH3 and its mechanism of action.

Dr. Aslan defined GH3 as procaine (the famous dental anesthetic),
stabilized with small amounts of benzoic acid, potassium meta-bisulfate,
and disodium phosphate. It is thought that GH3 (or its "cousin" KH3)
suppresses monoamine oxidase (MAO) levels. Elevated MAO interferes
with the neurotransmitters—dopamine and norepinephrine—and leads
to suppressed cortisol levels. In the 1970s, it was used as a drug for
treating depression because it effectively increases serotonin levels.

Other GH3/KH3 benefits reported in journals over the years include sta-bilizing brain cell membranes in ways that reverse "normal" age-related membrane deterioration; increasing general intracellular metabolic rate, especially in muscle cells; and increasing intracellular DNA levels necessary for optimal regeneration and repair of age-induced cellular "wear and tear."

Although the studies regarding the effects of GH3 were clinical trials involving thousands of elderly subjects, most researchers of the 1960s contradicted the so-claimed beneficial effects of the treatment devel-oped by Aslan (Ostfeld *et al.*, 1977). The negative outlook and backlash were caused because, at that time, Gerovital was more about market-ing as a "miraculous anti-aging product" than indisputable scientific evidence. In 1982, following the study commissioned by the National Institute on Aging, the U.S. Food and Drug Administration (FDA) banned GH3 for "anti-aging and associated claims" (Perls, 2013).

Centrophenoxine

Centrophenoxine is also known as "meclofenoxate." Developed in 1959, this molecule is composed of parachlorophenoxyacetate (PCPA) and dimethylaminoethanol (DMAE). The latter is a naturally occurring sub-stance that crosses the blood–brain barrier and acts in the brain. It facili-tates the synthesis of neurotransmitters involved in the transmission of nerve impulses. Centrophenoxine increases acetylcholine activity in the brain, enhancing general cognition and short-term memory. These func-tions naturally degrade with age, making this supplement for memory and brain function a potential game-changer.

Centrophenoxine has also shown potential for combatting free radi-cals inside the brain. These free radicals are caused by natural oxidation and heavy metal waste, a natural consequence of aging. Scientists have identified it as a powerful brain antioxidant, able to combat the oxidative stress responsible for the aging of the brain. More specifically, studies have found that it affects lipofuscin, a metabolic waste product associ-ated with aging, the accumulation of which alters brain cell function and disrupts the transmission of nerve impulses to organs. Some studies also suggest centrophenoxine stimulates brain function. While its pre-cise mechanisms of action are not yet fully understood, it seems it im-proves the brain's use of glucose and oxygen. Yet, despite the claims for increasing brain function, we could not find any published studies on increasing longevity.

Phosphatidylserine

Phosphatidylserine is one of the phospholipids present in cell membranes, especially in brain and the rest of the nervous system. Phosphatidylserine levels are reduced with aging, and this age-related decrease in phosphatidylserine is known to contribute to cognitive impairment and Alzheimer's disease. *Caenorhabditis elegans,* a nematode measuring about 1 mm in length, is a useful model for studying aging mutations and has been used to study this compound. A survey of the *C. elegans* genome indicates that this "simple" worm contains many genes with a high degree of similarity to human genes. There is a large body of scientific evidence that describes the interactions among cognitive activity, oxidative stress, neurodegeneration, neuroprotection, cognitive aging, and retention of cognitive functioning ability. Phosphatidylserine has been shown to increase life span in *C. elegans* (Kim & Park, 2020), but no studies have been published on humans.

Deprenyl

Deprenyl, marketed as "selegiline," is an anti-Parkinson's drug thought to have a neuroprotective effect, working by protecting neurons against a variety of neurotoxins. Deprenyl can also delay or block apoptosis—cell death—meaning that understanding and using it could bring longevity one step closer. In the 1980s, studies published in Europe (Knoll, 1988) showed remarkable life span increase in rats treated with the drug. Treatment at just 0.5 mg/kg increased life expectancy by 34% in 24-month-old rats.

The deprenyl-treated rats were also more mobile and sexually active. When the study was extended to dogs (giving a better indication of how the drug would work on humans), researchers discovered that dogs between the ages of 10 and 15 years treated with deprenyl, at 1 mg/kg, survived significantly longer than dogs in the placebo group, with 80% of treated dogs being alive at the time the study was published versus just 39% of placebo-treated dogs (Ruehl *et al.*, 1997). We are still waiting for a prospective, double-blind study in humans.

Acetyl-L-carnitine

Acetyl-L-carnitine (ALC) is the active form of the amino acid L-carnitine and has been shown to protect cells throughout the body against age-related degeneration. Beneficial effects include improved mood, memory, and cognition. By facilitating the youthful transport of fatty acids into the cell's mitochondria, ACL better enables dietary fats to be converted to energy and muscle. It is claimed to have effects on muscle-wasting diseases, such as cardiomyopathy, congestive heart failure, and chronic fatigue. It is also claimed to have effects on the immune system. The anti-aging effects, however, work with coenzyme Q10 and alpha lipoic acid to maintain the function of mitochondria. When the mitochondria function dwindles, degenerative disease becomes an inevitable consequence.

According to WebMD, ALC is sometimes used for Alzheimer's disease, improving memory and thinking skills, treating symptoms of depression, and reducing nerve pain in people with diabetes. It is used for many other conditions, but there is no good scientific evidence to support many of these uses.

There are many claims on the Internet that a substantial number of older patients use ALC for maintaining vitality and for brain and heart health. These patients also claim that ALC helps with mood, improves depression, and enhances libido for men. However, there are no published intervention studies using ALC to promote longevity.

Melatonin

Melatonin is a hormone that plays a role in sleep. The production and release of melatonin in the brain is connected to time of day, increasing when it's dark and decreasing when it's light. Melatonin production declines with age. Melatonin has been advocated for circadian rhythm sleep disorders in the blind, delayed sleep–wake phase disorder, insomnia, jetlag, shiftwork disorder, and sleep disorders in children.

Karasek (2004) discussed the need to search for any therapeutic agent that might improve the quality of life in the elderly and suggested a possible role for melatonin. The declining levels may affect many circadian rhythm disturbances. The hormone exhibits immunomodulatory properties, and a remodeling of immune system function is an integral part of aging. The deficiency may also result in reduced antioxidant protection in the elderly, which may have significance not only for aging per se but also may contribute to the incidence or severity of some age-related diseases. However, the conclusion was that there were not enough data to conclude that melatonin may have a role in extending normal longevity. Because melatonin is relatively inexpensive and is easily available, many "dedicated life extensionists" recommend taking melatonin even though there are no direct studies on its effect on longevity in humans.

Now, to the most interesting aspects of this chapter. There are beginning to appear novel ideas that have real science behind them. They include the use of the following:

- Very low-calorie diets
- Senolytic drugs
- Senomorphic drugs

We will explore each of those and share useful information with you.

Very Low-Calorie Diets

Chronic caloric restriction for increasing longevity is not new. In 1935, a scientist named Clive McCay (McDonald & Ramsey, 2010) published a startling discovery: Rats with severely calorie-restricted diets lived up to 33% longer than previously known possible. The health benefits of chronic caloric restriction resulting in life span extension are well established. Caloric restriction, that is, reducing calorie availability by 20% to 50%, is one of the rare known strategies that can extend life span. In short-lived species such as rodents, caloric restriction can increase maximal life span up to 50% while improving general health and decreasing aging-associated diseases (Fontana et al., 2010). Beneficial effects of caloric restriction on age-related diseases have also been reported for long-lived species, including rhesus monkeys and lemurs.

Why does caloric restriction (50% of normal) improve longevity? First, it is not overeating that is reduced; it is lowering the total consumption of food. There are two theories about aging that may apply: the rate of living theory and the free radical theory.

The rate of living theory can be best understood by the observation that larger animals tend to live longer than smaller ones. Elephants live longer than humans, which live longer than dogs, which live longer than rodents, which live longer than yeast. One explanation of that observation has to do with metabolic rate, how quickly an animal expends energy for the body's day-to-day functioning (breathing, maintaining body temperature, heart beating, and circulating blood). Larger animals have been observed to have lower metabolic rates. This suggests that slower metabolic rates are associated with longer life spans.

The free radical theory has been talked about for many years. Under this theory, aging is a result of damage in cells accumulating over time. The damage may be caused by "free radicals" that are highly reactive atoms or molecules naturally produced by our bodies. The theory is that they can damage proteins, DNA, and fatty tissue, which is theorized to cause age-related diseases such as heart disease, neurodegenerative disorders (Parkinson's disease, Alzheimer's disease, dementia), or cancer. Slower metabolism could decrease the rate of free radical production and subsequently extend life.

It is important to understand, however, that not all scientists accept those theories as the cause of aging. They may be part of the aging process, but there may be many other theories that may turn out to be true. The free radical theory is still extremely popular.

Caloric restriction will reduce metabolic rate. If there is less food (and calories) to process, the body has to work less. As a result of this reduction of metabolic rate, it is hypothesized that calorie restriction could extend life span by decreasing the rate of free radical damage. Unfortunately, there is no way to measure free radical damage, leaving some legitimate criticism of this theory.

Even though many studies in lower animals and rodents show positive results in life extension with calorie restriction, one must be a little skeptical about similar studies in humans, mainly because it is quite easy to control food consumption in laboratory animals and very difficult to control human food consumption when people are on their own. So, there are very few studies in humans. The one study that is often quoted is the CALERIE trial (Comprehensive Assessment of Long-term Effects of Reducing Intake of Energy) (Kraus et al., 2019). That study looked at 238 subjects, aged 21 to 50, non-obese people; half of them were in a calorie reduction group and the other half in a control group. Because the trial only lasted for two years, the effects on life span could not be directly measured, and the goal of the study was to investigate the effects on typical markers of age-related disease risk. The calorie restriction group was told to reduce caloric intake by 25%. Unfortunately, they only reduced their intake by 12%. Nevertheless, significant health benefits were observed even at 12% calorie intake. These include lower cholesterol and blood pressure levels, as well as improved insulin sensitivity. Unfortunately, this trial did not answer the question of whether metabolic changes due to calorie reduction can improve health. The trial was also too short to determine the long-term effects, good or bad.

More research is needed, and calorie restriction does seem promising, but it is too challenging for most people to follow for even a brief period of time.

Another small study (Wei et al., 2017) looked at fasting-mimicking diets practiced for 5 days a month for 3 months. Fasting decreased Basal Metabolic Rate (BMR), glucose, triglycerides, cholesterol, and C-reactive protein (a marker for inflammation). These effects were generally larger in the subjects who were at greater risk of disease at the start of the study. A larger study is needed to replicate these results, but they do raise the possibility that fasting may be a practical road to a healthy metabolic system.

This type of eating is something to consider because it makes sense, but it is very difficult to follow. This decision ultimately is yours. The same with intermittent fasting, no matter how that is carried out.

Senolytics and pro-longevity drugs

Senolytics may turn out to be very important in increasing longevity. "Senolytic" comes from the words "senescence" and "-lytic." They are a class of small molecules currently under research to determine if they can selectively induce death of senescent cells and improve health in humans (Childs et al., 2015). The goal of research is to discover or develop agents to delay, prevent, alleviate, or reverse age-related diseases (Kirkland & Tchkonia, 2015). Senomorphic drugs modulate properties of senescent cells without eliminating them, suppressing phenotypes of senescence.

Senolytic drugs are agents that selectively induce apoptosis (programmed cell death) of senescent cells. These cells accumulate in many tissues with aging and at sites of pathology in multiple chronic diseases. In studies in animals, targeting senescent cells using genetic or pharmacological approaches delays, prevents, or alleviates multiple age-related phenotypes, chronic diseases, geriatric syndromes, and loss of physiological resilience. Among the chronic conditions successfully treated by depleting senescent cells in preclinical studies are frailty, cardiac dysfunction, vascular hyperactivity and calcification, diabetes mellitus, liver steatosis, osteoporosis, and vertebral disk degeneration.

Mayo Clinic researchers (Kirkland & Zhu, 2022) say senolytic drugs can boost a key protein in the body that may protect older people against aspects of aging and a range of diseases. Senolytics clear the bloodstream of senescent or "zombie" cells. These cells contribute to multiple diseases and negative aspects of aging. This study shows that the removal of senescent cells significantly boosts the production of a protective protein called "α-Klotho." The protein α-Klotho is important to maintaining good health, as it tends to decrease with age, and especially decreases in multiple diseases, including Alzheimer's, diabetes, and kidney disease. Animal studies have shown that decreasing α-Klotho in mice shortens life span and increasing α-Klotho in mice by inserting a gene that causes its production increases life span by 30%. This study (Zhu et al., 2022) shows that senolytics, which can be administered orally, increase α-Klotho in humans with idiopathic pulmonary fibrosis, a senescence-associated disease that leads to frailty, serious breathing difficulties, and death.

There are many other senolytics that are in very early-stage human trials, including:

- FOXO4-related peptides
- Src inhibitors
- Quercetin+Dasatinib
- Navitoclax
- Navitoclax
- SSK-1
- QLS 1 inhibitors

- BCL-2 inhibitors
- USP-7 inhibitors
- Fisetin
- Piperlongumine
- Roxithromycin
- BIRC5 knockout
- Anti-GPNMB Vaccine

There are actually some products that claim to be senolytics that can now be purchased over the counter. They include the following:

- Format (Advanced Immune Support)
- Semolytic Activator
- Fesitin
- Activator-Senolytic Liposomal (Quercetin, Fisetin, Spermidine)
- Senolytic Complex
- GERO PROTECT Ageless Cell
- Immune Senescence Protection
- Qualia Semolytic

There are no long-term studies in humans with those products, although the ingredients in some of the above products are in early-stage clinical research.

If you want to find naturally occurring semolytics, some foods that contain quercetin, another semolytic, include green tea, coffee, berries, apples, onions, broccoli, citrus fruits, and red wine.

Senomorphic medications and pro-longevity medications

Senomorphic medications suppress the senescence-associated secretory phenotype (SASP) that drives sterile inflammation associated with aging to extend health span and potentially life span.

There are three molecules/compounds/medications that deserve special attention because so much has been written about them, and so much potential use has been anticipated.

- **NAD+**
- **Rapamycin**
- **Metformin**

NAD+ is a molecule that is present in all cells, central to more than 500 different metabolic reactions. It plays a key role in carbon metabolism and redox homeostasis. It is essential for life. That is, if we are deficient in our ability to synthesize or obtain NAD+, cells cannot survive. Because it impacts so many different aspects of cellular function, it is difficult to study. It is involved with the sharing of electrons, a process that is essential to life. Let's us explore how this molecule may work to prolong life.

NAD+ works through its interaction with the Sirtuin family of proteins. Sirtuins (Silent Information Regulators) are a family of seven proteins that help regulate the health of our cells. They are a group of enzymes that work to speed up certain chemical reactions in our bodies. Sirtuins are quite miraculous in the work they perform to manage the many processes in our cells that are involved in aging and the diseases associated with the aging processes. They are thought to be protectors for our cells. Supposedly, they:

- Support healthy DNA
- Are linked to the benefits of fasting and exercise
- Work with other genes and respond to damage in cells
- Make enzymes that work to control the epigenome
- Reduce the rate that cells divide
- Remove old decaying parts of our cells
- Sirtulins 3, 4, 5 work on the mitochondria
- Sirtulins 1, 5, 7 work on the nucleus
- Sirtulin 2 works on the cytoplasm

Sirtulins do not work on their own. They need the support of another molecule, NAD+. The intimate relationship between sirtulins and NAD+ is regulated at different levels allowing their coordinating role in metabolic processes, decreasing NAD+ availability due to aging, reducing sirtuins' activities, and affecting the communication between the nucleus and mitochondria. If we can increase NAD+, then we can theoretically activate sirtuins to become more vigorous in their work.

There are natural sources of NAD+ (kale, red wine, onions, soy, parsley, extra virgin olive oil, dark chocolate, turmeric, blueberries, and coffee). Functional foods and nutraceuticals/dietary ingredients are a great promise for health and longevity promotion and prevention of age-related chronic diseases.

The potent sirtuin-activating compounds (STACs) include:

- Favones, stilbenes, chalcones, and anthocyanidins that directly activate SIRT1
- Resveratrol
- Cilostazol
- Paeonol
- Statins
- Hydrogen sulfide
- Persimmon

However, the real questions are related to NAD+ itself. NAD+ is not something that can be taken orally. Intravenous form may not get into a cell. Therefore, active NAD+ precursors, such as nicotinamide riboside (NR) and nicotinamide mononucleotide (NMN), do get transported into the cell. Scientists are now studying these precursors in the context of aging. The real questions that need to be answered are—do these molecules have an effect on NAD levels, and do we see functional improvements in those cells and tissues?

The precursors, NR and NMN, are orally bioavailable, are safe from acute toxicity, and are available as over-the-counter supplements. Unfortunately, many experiments in mice do not increase life span. Also, it is not clear whether NAD+ levels should be elevated in the blood or in the tissue. There are mouse models of high level of DNA damage where there is depletion of NAD. In those mice, NR seems to work well in improving function and survival.

If the precursors are going to work, they probably have to be given in much higher doses. In doing that, you might overextend the capacity of the cells to buffer the NAD+. Who knows what complications of that might occur and in which cells? Even though one study did show a very slight improvement in delaying the progression of ALS, it is far from enough to justify the use of these precursors right now to prolong life span.

Metformin is a medicine used together with diet to lower high blood sugar levels in patients with type 2 diabetes. Metformin works by lowering the amount of glucose absorbed from intestines, decreasing how much glucose is made in the liver, and improving insulin sensitivity. The first studies with this drug came from earlier studies in the 1980s by a Russian scientist named Vladimir Anisimov (2013) who was working with phenformin, a precursor of metformin. He proposed that biguanides (of which phenformin and metformin are examples) affect fatty acid metabolism which in some way is relevant for aging. He conducted some experiments showing that metformin extended life span in those mice. Right about that time, metformin was becoming a popular drug for treatment of patients with type 2 diabetes. Epidemiological studies in people with type 2 diabetes who were taking metformin appeared to live longer than other patients with the same disease who were taking other forms of treatment. However, one subsequent study showed that patients taking a high dose of metformin for diabetes treatment had a shorter life span than those patients taking a lower dose.

Metformin has been used to treat a variety of other diseases, including COVID-19. In polycystic ovary syndrome, metformin improves insulin sensitivity. In type 1, diabetes metformin may help reduce the insulin dose. Meta-analysis and data from preclinical and clinical studies link metformin to a reduction in the incidence of cancer. Preclinical and clinical data suggest that metformin, via suppression of pro-inflammatory pathways, protection of mitochondria and vascular function, and direct actions on neuronal stem cells, may protect against neurodegenerative diseases. Metformin has also been studied for its antibacterial, antiviral, and anti-malaria efficacy. It remains unclear as to whether these beneficial effects are secondary to its actions as an anti-hyperglycemic and insulin-sensitizing drug, or result from other cellular actions, including inhibition of mTOR (mammalian target for rapamycin, see below), or direct antiviral actions. Clinical trials, including MILES (Metformin in Longevity Study) and TAME (Targeting Aging with Metformin), have been designed to determine if metformin can offset aging and extend life span. These studies are ongoing. TAME is still recruiting patients.

We still do not know how metformin works. It might activate cyclic AMP kinase. It might be an electron transport chain inhibitor. It might affect folate metabolism in the microbiome. It could be acting through all those paths or even others, all at the same time. At this time, with the information we know, metformin should be used for people who are insulin-resistant, especially those who are unable or unwilling to do intense exercise.

Rapamycin is a macrocyclic lactone antibiotic, secreted by the bacterium *streptomyces hygroscopicus* that was discovered on the Easter Island in 1972 (Tee, 2018). It was originally intended for use as an antifungal agent. However, its immunosuppressive and antiproliferative properties rendered it unsuitable as a safe antifungal treatment. Instead, these properties of rapamycin led to its development for other purposes, and rapamycin, along with its derivatives, are FDA-approved for use as immunosuppressants and as an anticancer agent (Lamming *et al.*, 2013).

Rapamycin or one of its derivatives has been used for treatment of a very rare condition called "Hutchinson-Gilford Progeria Syndrome" (progeria). Children with progeria show early signs of aging, which include loss of body fat and hair, growth failure, stiffness of joints, aged-looking skin, hip disloca-tion, cardiovascular disease, stroke, and generalized atherosclerosis. The life span of children with HGPS is 14 years, with the common cause of death being atherosclerosis. Thus, the correlation between HGPS and normal ag-ing suggests rapamycin as a possible drug to promote longevity in the gen-eral population (Graziotto *et al.*, 2012).

In 2009, a study showing that rapamycin extended the life span of mice was published (Harrison *et al.*, 2009). This was the first study to realize the anti-aging properties of rapamycin on mammals. Since then, rapamycin has been explored as a possible anti-aging drug for humans.

Blagosklonny (2019) wrote an opinion in 2019. He reviewed the history of rapamycin and the use of it as an antibacterial, antiviral, and immune modulator. He also reviewed the clinical data on the use of HGH and anti-oxidants, which turned out not to be longevity-promoting. There are many scientists working independently all over the world who have demonstrated that rapamycin inhibits mTOR in diverse organisms, such as yeast, worms, and flies. Mammalian target of rapamycin (mTOR) regulates cell proliferation, autophagy, and apoptosis by participating in multiple signaling pathways in the body. It was predicted that conversion from quiescence to senescence (geroconversion) is derived by growth-promoting mediators, such as mTOR, when the cell cycle is blocked. In cell culture, mTOR is maximally activated, and geroconversion lasts 3 to 6 days, whereas in the human body, it may take decades. Because of these observations, researchers have studied ra-pamycin for the prevention and treatment of nearly every age-related dis-ease, including cancer, obesity, atherosclerosis, and neurodegeneration. If a drug is indicated for all age-related diseases, it must be an anti-aging drug in that it targets a common driver of age-related diseases. This is because ag-ing is the sum of all age-related diseases that limit life span. So, the question is, does rapamycin suppress aging and extend life span by preventing diseases, or does it prevent diseases by slowing aging? It may do both.

Blagosklonny (2019) felt that the overwhelming evidence suggests that rapamycin is a universal anti-aging drug. Even though it may reverse some manifestations of aging, it is most effective in slowing down aging than reversing it. Therefore, it should be most effective when administered at the pre-disease or pre-pre-disease stages of age-related diseases. He even advocates the anti-aging "cocktail" of rapamycin, metformin, aspirin, angiotensin-converting enzyme (ACE) inhibitors, angiotensin receptor blockers (ARB), and PDES inhibitors, each of which can prevent or treat more than one age-related disease. All of those are clinically approved drugs, even if they have to be used off-label. Unfortunately, there are no short-term markers of anti-aging effects. Before taking rapamycin, researchers must be sure that the therapy is safe. In the future, the treatment should be conducted as a life-long phase I/II trial. If Blagosklonny is correct, treatment with rapamycin might need to be life-long unless discontinued due to side effects. These side effects include sore or inflamed mouth, weakened immune system, anemia and fatigue, constipation or diarrhea, elevated cholesterol or other lipid levels, high blood pressure, and swollen hands or feet.

He also cautioned that self-medication should be avoided and strongly discouraged. Instead, we need anti-aging centers that implement the entire anti-aging recipe, including diet and lifestyle changes. Blood levels of rapamycin should be monitored, and the dose of the medication tailored to each person.

Take-Home Information

The conclusion of all these observations, studies, and research is that the scientists are getting closer, but are still not there yet. Until the time comes when double-blind, controlled studies are available and published in scientific journals, all we have for our decision-making are the animal studies and personal feelings. Dr. Richard Miller at the Paul F. Glenn Center on Aging at the University of Michigan suggests that "within the next 10 years, we will know whether these drugs slow aging in dogs, and humans will come next."

Despite this lack of research and claims that it might take years to know the results on humans, many so-called longevity centers have appeared all over the country (see Appendix C). They each tend to recommend one or more of the products discussed above, or maybe others that we have not even mentioned. Our only comment is that you, our reader, should be careful wherever you go. Before you start taking any new product, including those you can buy yourself over the counter, on the Internet, from out of the country, sold to you at a center, and even those medications that are used "off-label" (meaning approved by the FDA for one condition, but used for a totally different condition), think twice whether there is any value in what you are about to do. These products may be naturally occurring substances, but they are bioactive even though they are not necessarily approved by the FDA. Side effects can and do occur. You might have to do your own due diligence to find out what side effects might occur, especially if no one warns you in advance.

Last, be careful whom you turn to for advice. Most health care providers are not knowledgeable about anti-aging therapy. Some of the clinics that are out there may be run by physicians, some of whom are certified by some type of accrediting agency. It is very important to keep in mind that you try to vet the person who gives you advice. Ask about his or her education, including medical school, residency, fellowships, and other courses taken or certifications obtained. This information may be on the website of the clinic. Make sure you ask about which medications (treatments, infusions, supplements, or vitamins) are being prescribed and why. Then ask about any published studies on humans that are the basis for the prescription. Last, ask about the success of that provider in using a particular product and how many patients have they treated with the product. If the provider only gives you anecdotal reports from previous clients, and no real statistics, like "I used this product on ___ patients, ages ___ to ___. I followed them for ___ months or years on average. ___% have died; ___% had complications; ___% are continuing to come back or at least communicating with me from afar." If you are satisfied with the response, then it is your choice. Also, know ahead of time, how much the program will cost. Do not be surprised if the initial consultation is $3,000 to $10,000 and the ongoing treatment can be $5,000 per year or more, depending on the products used. None of this should be covered by health insurance, except for any laboratory tests that are ordered.

What else can you do?

There are many other attempts at extending human lives, most of which are considered totally experimental and have not even been recruiting humans into clinical trials. This research is currently going on in academic and private institutions; however, none have reached the point of being available for human use.

Chemicals that are intended to slow down the aging process include sirtuin-activating polyphenols, such as resveratrol (Kaeberlein, 2010) and pterostilbene (McCormack & McFadden, 2013), and flavonoids, such as quercetin and fisetin (Martel *et al.*, 2020). Other popular supplements with even fewer biological pathways targeting aging include lipoic acid, curcumin, and Coenzyme Q10. Even low doses of ethanol as a potential supplement have been studied. All of these have yet to be reported as prolonging human life.

Nanotechnology shows promise in life extension by cell-repair machines being miniaturized and being inserted into cells. This is only a theoretical model. Cloning and body part replacements are certainly being worked on presently. Joints and limbs hold the most promise. Brain transplantation in primates failed miserably because of rejection. The use of human stem cells is discussed in Chapter 8 of this book. The source of stem cells still has to be worked out, and the way to manipulate these stem cells into doing what the scientists want them to do is still quite experimental. Replacement of body organs such as a mechanical heart or a mechanical pancreas and kidney do hold promise but are not just yet ready for large-scale use. The concept of cryonics, or low-temperature freezing ($-320°$ F), of a corpse until such time a cure for the terminal event that caused the person to die has been discussed but deemed a quackery. Combining techniques is certainly a possibility for the future, including removing aging cells and the use of telomere-lengthening machinery. Lysosomal hydrolases are discussed but are far from clinical trials. Genome editing in which pieces of DNA are delivered as a drug to create proteins, interfere with the expression of proteins, or to correct genetic mutations have all been proposed, but are not a reality, as yet. In 2020, scientists looked at data on nearly 2 million people and identified 10 genomic loci that appear to influence life span and longevity, of which half had not been reported previously, and most associated with premature cardiovascular disease. These sites are currently being investigated. Last, some clinics currently offer injections of blood products from young donors. The alleged benefits of this treatment have not been demonstrated in any randomized clinical studies. But their claims include not only longer life, darker hair, better memory, better sleep, but also no heart disease, diabetes, or Alzheimer's disease (Maxmen, 2017). Young blood does not reverse aging in mice, and those who offer those treatments have misunderstood the basic science research behind this procedure. For the record, two clinics in California still offer $8,000 injections of plasma extracted from the blood of young people. The leaders of the clinics have not published their results in any peer-reviewed journal (Foley, 2017).

If you are serious about these types of treatments, consider going to a longevity center associated with a major medical center. The list of those centers is quite long. Below are a few, although neither of us have visited them or spoken to their directors. The physicians at those types of centers tend to be more scientific about what they prescribe, but there is no guarantee that your outcome will be any better. Our deep apologies to any centers that we left off our list. That is no reflection of their quality or clinical successes.

State	City	Program
AL	Tuscaloosa	Alabama Research Institute on Aging
AZ	Tucson	Arizona Center of Aging at the University of Arizona Zuckerman College
CA	Los Angeles	UCLA Longevity Center
CA	Palo Alto	Stanford Center on Longevity
CO	Denver	Multidisciplinary Center of Aging at Anschutz Medical Campus, University of CO
IL	Chicago	Potocsnak Longevity Institute at Northwestern University Feinberg School of Medicine
MA	Boston	Harvard Center for Population and Development Studies
MD	Baltimore	Center on Aging and Health at Johns Hopkins University
MI	Ann Arbor	Paul F. Glenn Center for Aging Research at the University of Michigan
NC	Durham	Duke Aging Center
NJ	Princeton	Princeton Longevity Center
NY	NY	International Longevity Center at Columbia University
PA	Philadelphia	University of Pennsylvania Institute on Aging
PA	Pittsburgh	GERI Longevity Center of the University of Pittsburgh
TN	Nashville	Center for Quality Aging at Vanderbilt University Medical Center
WA	Seattle	University of Washington Healthy Aging and Longevity Research Institute

The last suggestion for you to consider—if you want to try one of the newer products (such as NAD+, metformin, rapamycin), you might consider participating in a clinical trial. These are research studies performed under very strict guidelines, usually at a major medical center.

You can find information about these studies on the government's website: www.clinicaltrials.org. Look for FIND A STUDY and then find the box CONDITION OR DISEASE. Type in "longevity." Look for a study in which you would like to participate. Then explore the site and find a center where you can go to enroll.

Here are some of the relevant studies listed, as of August 2022. This list changes often.

- Fitness and Longevity in Exercise
- Metformin and Longevity Genes in Prediabetes
- Metformin and Longevity
- Metformin in Longevity Study (MILES)
- Participatory Evaluation (of) Aging (with) Rapamycin (for) Longevity Study (PEARL)
- Safety and Efficacy of Extended Longevity Protocol
- Targeting Aging with Metformin (TAME)

As with all concepts in this book, our goal is just to present you with information to consider. We are not recommending any specific center or any specific type of intervention. Those decisions are always up to you.

APPENDIX A

Going Out to Dinner

Most Baby Boomers are retired or are nearly so. For many of us, cooking at home for two or maybe one person is not a viable option. Entertaining at home is often not worth the time and effort, unless one individual is really into shopping, preparation, cooking, and cleaning up. That is why going out to dinner almost every night is a given for many Baby Boomers. Not only is it easier than shopping, cooking, and cleaning; it is also a time for socialization, something we all need and enjoy. Looking forward to being with friends is a great opportunity to spend an evening together. Restaurants acknowledge that going out to dinner competes with other forms of entertainment, such as theater, concerts, lectures, and socializing in one's home. Nowadays, that is even more true, as many couples go out to dinner nearly every night, and making plans for dinner has become a major issue in life. Choosing the right restaurant, selecting the proper time, and often even sitting at the right table can be a very time-consuming set of details, yet that has become an important part of some people's lives. In addition, a study was presented at the annual meeting of the American Heart Association by Lora Burke (Burke, 2017), a professor of nursing at the University of Pittsburgh that showed what most people have suspected for years that going out to eat is a major risk for abandoning any diet or healthy eating plan. Another study (Urban *et al.,* 2016) showed that a staggering 92% of meals from large-chain and local restaurants had more than the recommended calories for the average person for a single meal. Some meals even exceeded the calories recommended for an entire day.

Now, the challenging part. If we are trying to make a change in our lives in an effort to become healthier and live longer, what should we eat when we go out to a restaurant for dinner? As you progress, you will quickly realize that a night at a restaurant can be a food-and-beverage challenge. As part of our mission to make suggestions of what you can do to live longer, we have decided to help you by sharing with you a look at menus from many different American and ethnic restaurants, including many that you might have frequented. We will look at menus from many different restaurants and suggest what you might order when you choose to go there. Once you see our comments, you will realize that going out to dinner is indeed a real challenge, and one that you should not wait to think about until the time when you have that menu in front of you. In many books about health, nearly half of the text in the books is composed of recipes. If you, however, are like most of us and go out to dinner nearly every night, this section can become a "bible" for you to follow. After we review the "generic" American and ethnic restaurants, we will provide you menus from some very popular sites in many cities for you to use as a guideline. Remember, most Italian, Japanese, Chinese, Mexican, and so on, restaurants serve similar dishes, but just prepared differently, depending on the chef. We thought that having specific menus to look at would be fun. Be prepared, Brian has a very critical eye, and he just might put your favorite place on the "Do not go to" list. Enjoy!

As you read through the menu items of each restaurant, including those that might be considered elegant, fast-food, casual dining, and even convenience stores, you will be able to see how unhealthy restaurant food can be. If the reason you are going out to dinner with friends is to socialize, try not to sabotage yourself by choosing a place where there is nothing healthy for you to eat. You might even consider getting in the habit of looking at menus online before you go so you can think about the choices you have, and you will not be forced into ordering food that is not healthy for you. During the COVID-19 Pandemic, most restaurants offered online ordering and food delivery. Most of those restaurants still maintain their menus on their websites.

The menus we provide here were all obtained from the websites of restaurants. With your new "critical eye," you can look carefully at exactly what is there to order. Do not be surprised now why there is such an epidemic of childhood obesity as there is an overt lack of healthy choices at most fast-food restaurants where some families tend to frequent. We have highlighted in gray our suggestions. It is still up to you to place the order.

As you read through the menus of all the restaurants, keep in mind how difficult it is to find healthy choices, even at the most widely patronized places, including those which may be on the pricey side. Also, keep in mind that restaurant-sized portions are often quite large, and eating too much at one meal is often just as deleterious as eating the wrong foods.

Types of American and Ethnic Restaurants

American	Israeli
Argentinian	Italian
Barbecue	Japanese
Brazilian	Mexican
Chinese	Pizza
Continental	Russian
Cuban	Seafood
Delicatessen	Spanish
Egyptian	Steak House
Ethiopian	Thai
French	Turkish
Greek	Vegan
Hamburger	Vegetarian
Indian	

Fast-Food Restaurants

Arby's	KFC
Burger Fi	McDonald's
Burger King	Popeye's
Chick-fil-A	Shake Shack
Chipotle Mexican Grill	Sonic Drive-In
Church's chicken	Starbucks
Einstein Brothers	Subway
Jamba Juice	Taco Bell
Jersey Mike's Subs	Wendy's
Long John Silvers	

Other Casual Dining Restaurants

Benihana	Legal Sea Foods
Bonefish Grill	Longhorn Steakhouse
Cheesecake Factory	Olive Garden
Chuck E. Cheese	Outback Steakhouse
Cracker Barrell	PF Chang China Bistro
Denny's	Red Lobster
Hard Rock Café	Seasons 52
Houston's	Sizzler
IHOP	TGI Fridays
J Alexander	

Convenience Store Takeouts

7-Eleven   Wawa

   There are now websites, like www.happycow.com (also available as a cell-phone app), which guides you to restaurants that contain options that are vegan, vegetarian, or have vegan options.

   As you scroll through all the restaurants, remember you can always ask your server if the chef or cook can modify a dish to meet your needs. An example might be to avoid sauces on top of food or ask for salad dressing to be delivered on the side. Another might be to ask if soups or vegetables are prepared in chicken or beef broth or contain ham or other animal products. You will find that getting in the habit of asking what you want is very well received.

American restaurant: Miami, FL

Appetizers
Mac n' cheese
Fried green tomatoes
Crispy Brussels sprouts
Buttermilk marinated chicken fingers
Bacon-wrapped and Gorgonzola-stuffed
   dates

Shrimp and grits
Duroc baby back ribs
House-made chips
Avocado salsa
Shrimp mac n' cheese

Salads
House (walnuts, cheese, tomatoes, raisins)
Fried chicken and organic spinach salad

Turkey cranberry
Skirt steak salad

Sandwiches
Tuna melt
Turkey and brie sandwich
Open-faced fried chicken BLT sandwich
Blackened chicken sandwich
Fried green tomato sandwich
Mozzarella Caprese sandwich
Skirt steak sandwich

BBQ pulled pork sandwich
Grilled cheese sandwich
Gourmet Southern pulled pork burrito
Chicken burrito
Steak burrito
Fish burrito
Vegetable burrito (without dairy)

Entrees
Full rack baby back ribs
Roasted ½ chicken
Spicy seared skirt steak
BBQ pork ribeye
Steak and potatoes
Shrimp and grits

Fried chicken breast
Roasted butterflied snapper
Bourbon and brown sugar seared salmon
Pan-seared Covina
Fried Mahi-Mahi sandwich
Pan-seared striped bass

Desserts
Bread pudding
Red velvet cake

Vanilla cheesecake
Key lime pie

Recommendations:
   Appetizer: Crispy Brussels sprouts
   Salad: Avocado salad
   Entrée: Vegetable burrito
   Dessert:
   Overall: ☐ 🔥 ☑ 🌱

Argentinian restaurant: Normandy Isle, FL

Appetizers and salads

Empanada (meat, chicken, or spinach)

Hearts of palm with pink sauce

Prosciutto or sweet ham with melon

Stuffed tomatoes (without dairy)

Boiled shrimp with hearts of palm

Russian salad (potatoes, carrots, peas, mayo)

Carrots and boiled egg

Mussels Provencal

Veal with spinach, carrots, salad

Grilled Provolone cheese

Boiled shrimp with pink sauce

Sliced Spanish raw ham

Lettuce, tomatoes, and onions

Beets and boiled eggs

Entrees

Breaded chicken

Breaded chicken with fried eggs

Eggplant with tomato and cheese

Grilled Provolone cheese

Grilled sausage

Thin rolled sausage

Fillet mignon

Blood sausage

Sweetbreads

Entrails

Flap meat

Rolled veal

Rolled steak

Boneless chicken breast

Sides

French fries

Fried sweet potatoes

Mashed potatoes

Mashed potatoes with garlic

Spinach sauté

Spinach, cauliflower, broccoli and carrots

Grilled red pepper

Pastas

Spaghetti

Fettuccine

Ravioli with spinach

Ravioli with meat

Sandwiches

Skirt steak

Blood sausage

Breaded chicken

Sweetbreads

Desserts

Flan

Tiramisu

Recommendations:	
Appetizer:	Heart of palm (order without pink sauce)
Salad:	Lettuce, tomato, onions
Entrée:	Order only sides: spinach, cauliflower, broccoli, carrots
Dessert:	
Overall:	☐ 👍 ☑ 👎

Barbecue restaurant: Kansas City, MO

Sandwiches

Beef

Pork

Sausage

Combo

Ham

Turkey

Burned ends

Specialty items

Baby back ribs

Half chicken

Side orders

French fries

Baked beans

Onion rings

Nothing is available to choose.

Recommendations:
    Appetizer:
    Salad:
    Entrée:
    Dessert:
    Overall: ☐ 👍 ☑ 👎

Brazilian restaurant: New York City, NY

Appetizers

Salad (arugula, spinach, seeds)

Cheese bread

Yuca fries

Sopa de Galinha

Caldinho de feijao

Amazon salad (no meat)

Coxinha

Tuna tartare

Mussels

Acai Bowl

Sides

Yuca puree

Creamy spinach

Beans

Rice

Collard greens

Caramelized banana

Farofa

Vinaigrette

Mains

Galinhada (organic chicken, black rice, baby carrots, grilled lemon, breadcrumbs)

Vegan Stroganoff (vegan hearts of palm, mushrooms, carrots, chickpeas, sweet peppers, quinoa, rice)

Chicken Stroganoff (chicken, mushrooms, garlic, cream, tomato, crispy potato sticks, rice)

Picanha Tom Jobim (pork, carrots, tomato, vinaigrette, farofa, rice, beans)

Vegan Feijoada (black bean stew, mushrooms, carrots, tofu, collard greens, orange, rice, farofa)

Arroz de pato (duck breast, spiced homey and cachaca glaze, rice with duck confit, smoked sausage, duck jus, frisee salad, orange puree)

Bobo de camarão (shrimp, coconut milk, onion, bell peppers, cassava, rice, farofa)

Fillet mignon Stroganoff (beef tenderloin, mushrooms, garlic, cream, tomato, crispy potato sticks, rice)

Mosquera banana

Feijoada (bean stew, pork, collard greens, orange rice, farofa)

Picanha burger (hamburger, fontina cheese, tomato, pickles, lettuce, aioli, yuca fries, brioche)

Milanese (crispy chicken, arugula salad, aioli)

Skirt steak

Desserts

Brigadeiro (chocolate fudge, chocolate cachaca, whipped cream)

Pudim de Leite (caramel flan, berries)

Recommendations:

    Appetizer:

    Salad: Arugula, spinach, seeds, or Amazon salad

    Entrée: Vegan stroganoff

    Dessert:

    Overall: ☑ 👍 ☐ 👎

Chinese restaurant San Francisco, CA

Dim Sum
Steamed BBQ pork
Shrimp dumpling
Savory vegetable dumpling
Phoenix tail prawn
Pork potsticker
Scallion cake
Pan-fried chicken bun
Seafood basil dumpling
Steamed spareribs
Snow pea shoots dumpling
Spinach dumpling (vegan)

Pork and shrimp Siu Mai
Chicken and mushroom dumpling
Stuffed lotus leaf
Crab claw
Chicken spring roll
Curried shrimp wonton
Mandarin dumpling
Scallop Siu Mai
Bean curd roll
Mushroom dumpling

Noodles and Rice
Rice noodle soup with shrimp
Egg noodle soup with shrimp
Long-life noodles (vegetarian)
Chicken chow mein

Rice noodle soup with BBQ pork
Egg noodle soup with BBQ pork
BBQ pork fried rice
Steamed rice

Sides and Specials
Sichuan chicken
Scallop balls on skewer
Turnip cake
Crisp tofu (vegetarian)
Eggplant with Hunan sauce

Salt and pepper pork
Chicken satay
Sautéed string beans with dried shrimp
Snap peas (chilled) with chile soy sauce
Chinese broccoli

Desserts
Egg custard tart
Mango pudding (only if non-dairy)

Sesame ball
Orange Jell-O

Be careful when ordering dumplings as some may include egg which you might choose
to avoid.

Recommendations:
    Appetizer: Spinach dumplings
    Salad: Lifelong noodles (vegetarian)
    Entrée: Snap peas
    Dessert:
    Overall: ☑ 👍 ☐ 👎

Continental restaurant: Atlanta, GA

Appetizers

Charcuterie and cheese selection

Baby arugula salad, nuts, cheese, vinaigrette

Jumbo lump crab cake, slaw, honey

Oysters on the half shell

Smoked salmon

White shrimp toast, jicama, pineapple

Exotic mushroom soup

Marinated golden and red beet salad, goat cheese

Peppercorn crusted kangaroo, lentils, bacon

Blue hill bay mussels

Baby kale salad, radicchio, chile

Entrees

Grilled Bay of Fundy salmon, potato arrugadas

Gulf red snapper, butternut squash risotto

Maple-marinated duck breast, ancient grain, rice

Cocoa-crusted corvina venison, sweet potato

Beef tenderloin, whipped potatoes

Roasted heritage pork chop, apple, polenta

Slow-braised rabbit, celery root

Roasted Springer Mountain chicken, cauliflower

Potato-crusted Georges Bank Cod

Wood-grilled Boz beef tenderloin, potato

Duck n' beef burger, sunny-side egg, spinach

Desserts

Flat White, chiffon, Dulce, ice cream

South-style pistachio pie

Guava sorbet pineapple

Strawberry chocolate mousse

Popcorn ice cream sundae

Spice cookie cheesecake

Guava sorbet pineapple

Recommendations:
    Appetizer:
    Salad: Arugula salad or baby kale salad
    Entrée:
    Dessert:
    Overall: ☐ 🔥 ☑ 🌱

Cuban restaurant: Tampa, FL

Salads
Chicken salad
Special house salad (without meat)
Fried green plantains

Appetizers
Ham croquettes
Yuca fries
Corn tamale

Entrees
Palomilla steak
Breaded steak
Ribeye steak grilled
Spanish beef stew
Grilled beef liver
Ground beef in sauce
Yellow rice and chicken
Breaded chicken breast
Breaded fish fillet
Tilapia fish fillet in garlic sauce
Fried shrimp

Milanesa steak with cheese
T-bone steak, grilled
Sautéed beef tenderloin
Roast eye round stuffed
Grilled or fried pork chops
Stuffed plantain
Baked chicken, white meat
Chicken napolitana with ham
Breaded fish fillet Russian style
Rice with squid chunks
Grilled salmon

Sides
Chicken soup
Red beans
Yellow rice
Moro rice
Fried ripe plantains
Yucca (if not fried)

Black bean soup (only vegetarian)
Spanish bean soup
White rice
French fries
Salad

Desserts
Sweet rice pudding
Cream cheese flan
Guavashell with cream cheese

Custard pudding
Bread pudding
Carrot cake

Recommendations:
  Appetizer:
  Salad: House salad
  Entrée: Bean soup, only if vegetarian
  Dessert:
  Overall: ☐ 👍 ☑ 👎

Delicatessen restaurant: New York City, NY

Appetizers
Bisco fries

Loaded potato pancake

Avocado toast

Classic buffalo wings

Homemade chicken tenders

Fried calamari

Fried shrimp

Chopped liver

Soups
Matzoh ball soup

Split pea soup (without meat or dairy)

Salads
Garden salad

Caesar salad

Greek salad (without cheese)

Scoop salad

BBQ chicken salad

Cobb salad

Entrees
Reuben sandwich

Pastrami Reuben sandwich

Corned beef sandwich

Pastrami sandwich

Brisket sandwich

Roasted turkey sandwich

Virginia ham sandwich

Hungarian Beef Goulash

Roasted half chicken

Shrimp parmigiana

Chicken parmigiana

Broiled salmon fillet

Tuna salad sandwich

BLT

Chicken salad sandwich

Egg salad sandwich

Grilled cheese sandwich

Chopped liver sandwich

Club sandwich

Brisket platter

Roast turkey

Romanian tenderloin sandwich

Broiled cod fillet

Fish and chips

Sides
Red skin potato salad

Steak cut French fries

Batter dipper onion rings

Creamy cold slaw

Mashed potato

Macaroni and cheese

Recommendations:
    Appetizer:
    Salad: Garden salad
    Entrée: Split pea soup, only if vegetarian
    Dessert:
    Overall: ☐ 🔥 ☑ 🌱

Egyptian restaurant: Houston, TX

Appetizers
Baba ghanoush
Yogurt cucumber salad
Tabouli salad
Labneh with Za'atar
Kibbeh (deep-fried wheat stuffed
    with beef)
Appetizers

Stuffed grape leaves
Shrimp scampi
Mixed Vege (hummus, baba genus, tabouli)
Falafel

Salads
Caesar salad
Greek salad
Garden salad

Soups
Lentil soup if vegetarian
Chicken soup
Molokhia soup
Kawara'a soup

Entrees
Beef shish kabob
Talapia fish fillet
Mixed Grill (chicken, beef,
    and kufta kabob)
Hummus
Beef Shawarma
Beef Shawarma sandwich
Sambusa (meat, cheese, pasterma,
    sausage)
Macaroni Bashamel (beef and beshamel
    sauce)
Koshari ultimate veggie dish (rice, lentils,
    chickpeas, tomato sauce, fried onions)

Chicken shish kabob
Kofta shish kabob
Lamb shish kabob

Chicken Shawarma
Grilled quail
Falafel platter
Danadanah steak

Lamb chops

Seafood platter

Jumbo shrimp

Sides
French fries
Rice

Mixed pickles
Fresh bread

Recommendations:
    Appetizer: Tabouli salad
    Salad: Garden salad
    Entrée: Koshari ultimate veggie dish
    Dessert:
    Overall: ☑ 👍 ☐ 👎

Ethiopian restaurant: Washington, D.C.

Appetizers
Sambusa with veggie (pastry shell with lentils)

Sambusa with meat

Dukem salad

Entrees
Regular TIBS (beef and onion)

Awaze TIBS

Regular Kitfo (beef tartare)

Ze!!! Kitfo (beef with sliced onion, jalapeno)

Dullet (charred lamb)

Gored TIBS

Goden TIBS

Duken Kitfo (beef tartare + cottage cheese)

Gored (cubed meat)

Vegetarian Dishes
Veggie combo (lentil, peas, greens, salad)

Yesom Kulet Fitfit (veggie stew on bread)

Veggie combo (lentil, peas, greens, cabbage, etc.)

Other Dishes
Lamb Wot (stew)

Minchet Abesh (beef in ginger and garlic sauce)

Doro Wot (chicken stew)

Melasena Semba (beef and tongue in ginger sauce)

Desserts
Teramusso

White chocolate cake

Napoleon

Baklava

Recommendations:
    Appetizer: Sambusa with vegies
    Salad:
    Entrée: Veggie combo
    Dessert:
    Overall: ☑ 👍 ☐ 👎

French restaurant: Paris, France

Appetizers
Huitres (oysters)

Foie gras et volaille (foie gras and chicken)

Tartare de boeuf (fillet + caviar)

Homard a la Parisienne (whole lobster)

Poireaux vinaigrette (leeks, hazelnuts)

Thon a la portugaise (bigeye tuna tartar)

Lotte en salade au cumin (monkfish with cumin)

Entrees
Bar noir a la setoise (black sea bass, shrimp)

Halibut, beurre blanc (fermented daikon)

Legumes a la mode (veggies cooked like tripe)

Canette a l'Orange (duckling)

Fillet basquaise (prime fillet, foie gram and ham)

Homard Bourse et la Vie (lobster, sauce au poivre)

Sole Veronique (dover sole)

Tout le pain (rabbit)

Cote de veau Vallee d'Auge (veal)

Desserts
Millefeuille au gingembre (ginger + cream)

Baba au Rhum (chocolate tart, passion fruit)

Pavlova au paplemousse (meringue, sorbet)

Marjolaine (hazelnut dacquoise and cream)

Nothing to choose at this time.

Recommendations:
Appetizer:
Salad:
Entrée:
Dessert:
Overall: ☐ 👍 ☑ 👎

Greek restaurant: Chicago, IL

Appetizers

Spreads (taramosalata, melitzanosalata)
Melitzanosalata (eggplant, garlic, oil)
Skordalia (garlic-potato spread)
Hummus (chickpeas, tahini, spices)
Feta cheese (cheese + olive oil)
Sweet peppers (marinated in oil)
Saganaki (flaming cheese)
Grilled calamari
Homemade gyros
Fried zucchini
Spinach cheese pie
Hot lima beans

Taramosalata (Greek caviar)
Tzatziki (yogurt-cucumber-garlic spread)
Tirokafteri (feta cheese + peppers)
Kefalotiri (aged cheese)
Beets in olive oil

Grilled octopus
Homemade sausage
Mini pork kebobs
Eggplant in cheese
Dolmades (stuffed grape leaves)
Pita

Entrees

Gyros
Chicken reganati (with rice and potatoes)
Spartin chicken

Mousaka (eggplant, meat, and potato)
Dolmades (grape leaves, rice, ground
    meat)
Vegetarian shish kabob
Roast leg of lamb
Arni Fournou (lamb with potatoes)
Arni with spinach rice
Spaghetti (Greek-style pasta and cheese)
Rice and yogurt

Fresh whole fish
Broiled swordfish shish kabob
Shrimp tourkolimano
Souvlaki (pork tenderloin shish kabob)
Artichokes

Kontosouvli (pork on spit)
Mediterranean chicken breast
Veggie Mousake (eggplant, zucchini, and,
    potato)
Pasticcio (pasta, meat, cheese)
Vegetarian plate

Spanakotiropita (spinach and feta cheese)
Kokkinisto (lamb in tomato sauce)
Arni Aginarato (lamb with artichoke hearts)
Keftedes (beef and lamb meatballs)
Spaghetti with chicken breast
Spaghetti with vegetables

Broiled seafood shish kabob
Lake Superior white fish tail
Shrimp shish kabob
Homemade sausage
Fasolakia (baked string beans)

Recommendations:
  Appetizer: Spreads or hummus
  Salad: Hot lima beans
  Entrée: Vegetarian shish kabob or vegetarian plate
  Dessert:
  Overall: ☑ 👍 ☐ 👎

Hamburger restaurant: Omaha, NE

Appetizers
None

Entrees
Grass-fed black Angus beef burger
Grilled chicken burger
No hormone or GMO turkey burger
Thai black bean vegan burger
   (only no bun)

Cheese (American, cheddar, gouda, Swiss)
Extras (jalapenos, onion, mushrooms, slaw)
Sauce (ketchup, mayo, mustard, BBQ, aioli)
Bun (brioche, lettuce, white, sourdough)

Sides
Potatoes (hand cut, crinkle cut, curly)
Sweet potato fries

Crispy hashbrowns
New Orleans kettle-cooked chips

Children's menu
Kids slider
Chicken tenders and fries
Hotdogs and fries

Specialty Burgers, all with fries
BLT
Bold & Blazin'
Cheddar under Swiss
Clucker club
Gooey 3-cheese grilled cheese
Hello sunshine (beef sausage, cheese, egg)

Recommendations:
   Appetizer:
   Salad:
   Entrée:
   Dessert:
   Overall: ☐ 👍 ☑ 👎

Indian restaurant: Las Vegas, NV

Entrees
Kerelan pepper chicken
Kofta Shah Jahani
Coconut Cilanto Goan Kofta
Benarasi Mattar Ghugni

Bengali Kosha Mangsho
Murg Akbari
Chennai Express

Curries
Chicken Tikka masala
Butter chicken
Prawn masala
Fish Goa curry
Lamb or chicken vindaloo
Dal goshi

Chicken masala
Lamb or chicken korma
Fish masala
Rogan Josh
Dai children
Sag goshi

Vegetable Side Dishes
Spiced vegetable curry (cauliflower, beans, etc.)
Kali Dal New Delhi (black lentils)
Sag paneer (spinach, cheese, garlic)
Dhingri alu (mushrooms and potatoes)

Alu New Delhi (potato in tomato-cream sauce)
Malai kofta (cheese croquettes)

Palak kofta kashmiri (spinach stuffed with saffron)
Yellow dal tarka (yellow lentils, garlic, cumin)
Vegetable korma (cooked in coconut milk)
Sabzi Malabar (vegetables in yogurt-coconut milk)
Dum maro dum alu (poppy seeds, pancyphoram)
Navrattan curry (vegetables in cream and spices)

Rice and Breads
Lucknowi pullao (saffron-flavored rice)

Kashmiri pullao (saffron-flavored rice and fruit)
Indian fried rice (cooked with vegetables, eggs)
Garlic nan

Vegetable pullao (saffron rice and vegetables)
Pullao raja (saffron rice with vegetables and eggs)
Nan (soft bread)

Kabuli nan (with fruits and nuts)

Specialties
Chicken kofta kebab
Achari boti kebab (lamb)
Vegetable shashlyk (vegies, onions, potatoes)

Teengri kebab (chicken in yogurt, spices)
Fish tikka (salmon)
Bombay bhindi bhuna (okra, veg)

Recommendations:
　　Appetizer:
　　Salad:
　　Entrée:　　　Spiced vegetable curry or vegetable shashlyk
　　Dessert:
　　Overall:　　☑🖐 ☐👎

Israeli restaurant Philadelphia, PA

Appetizers

Laffa bread (Za'atar, olive oil)

Hummus-Tehina (green tehina)

Haloumi (kataifi, orange, urfa, pistachio)

Roasted broccolini (feta, spring onion,
    grapes)

Salatim (six vegetable salads)

Fried carrots (harissa honey, whipped feta)

Asparagus (chickpeas, labneh, ramps)

Entrees

Swordfish (pilpelchuma kale tzatzkik,
    orange)

Mushroom (freekeh, herbed tehina,
    sumac)

Cauliflower chraime (no African tomato
    stew)

Chicken shashlyk (muhammara , pickled
    celery)

Pomegranate lamb shoulder

Desserts

Coffee and hazel nut basboosa

Mango guava sorbet

Recommendations:

    Appetizer: Humus and techina
    Salad:
    Entrée: Mushrooms
    Dessert:
    Overall: ☑ 👍 ☐ 👎

Italian restaurant Providence, RI

Appetizers

Garlic bread

Fried zucchini

Fried calamari

Cold antipasto

Stuffed artichokes (without stuffing)

Baked clams

Stuffed mushrooms

Zupa di clams

Spicy scarpariello wings

Portobello parmigiana

Salads

Caesar salad

Mixed green salad

Seafood

Salmon oreganata

Shrimp scampi

Lobster fra diavolo

Shrimp marinara

Shrimp scampi

Broiled lobster oreganata

Pasta (only gluten free)

Garlic and oil

Penne alla vodka

Giardiniera

Marinara (without anchovy paste)

Pomodoro

Rigatoni and broccoli

Steaks

Broiled porterhouse steak

Porterhouse pizzailola

Sides

Sautéed broccoli

Sautéed escarole

Meatballs

Sautéed spinach

Eggplant parmigiana

Sweet Italian fennel sausage

Desserts

Chocolate torte

Bread pudding

Tiramisu

Italian cheesecake

Strawberry shortcake

Chocolate cannoli

Tartufi

Seasonal fruit platter

Recommendations:

Appetizer:	Stuffed artichoke
Salad:	Mixed green salad
Entrée:	Gluten-free pasta with garlic/oil or pomodoro sauce
Dessert:	Seasonal fruit platter
Overall:	☑ 👍 ☐ 👎

Japanese restaurant: Los Angeles, CA

Appetizers

Miso soup
Sunomono (cucumber and seaweed)
Asparagus goma ae (sesame sauce)
Takenoko tosa ae (bamboo with bonito
   and soy)
Wakasagi nanbanzuke (fried shellfish)
Komochi yari ika (squid)

Edamame
Spinach ohitashi (marinated with soy)
Ginnan (fried ginkgo nuts)
Seaweed salad

Hama sui (clear soup with clams)
Noresore (baby sea eel)

Sushi

Fresh abalone
Salmon
Yellowtail
Spanish mackerel
Japanese Spanish mackerel
Amberjack
Japanese barracuda
Squid
Seared bonito
Seared king mackerel
Firefly squid
Seared bonito
Blue fin tuna

Loupe de mar
Dorado
Fresh water eel
Fresh sardine
French snapper
Red snapper
Grouper
Shad
Seared Japanese barracuda
Striped jack
Shad
Seared Japanese halibut fin
Fresh squid

Hand rolls

Cucumber
Salmon skin
Spicy tuna
Salmon
Fresh water eel
California roll
Minced toro with green onions (tuna belly)
Soft shell crab roll

Vegetable
Spicy cod with roe
Yellowtail with Scanlon
Shrimp tempura
Blue crab
Tuna
Minced toro with pickled radish (tuna belly)

Recommendations:
   Appetizer: Miso soup or edamame or asparagus with sesame sauce
   Salad: Seaweed salad
   Entrée: Hand rolls or vegetable rolls
   Dessert:
   Overall: ☑ 🔥 ☐ 🌡

Mexican restaurant: San Antonio, TX

Appetizers

Guacamole en molcajete

Guacamole with bacon and cheese

Crispy shrimp with chile

Nachos with cheese, black beans, guacamole

Quesadilla, if vegetarian

Caesar salad

Chopped salad (no egg or cheese)

Ceviche (tuna)

Guacamole with pineapple pico de gallo

Guacamole with crab meat

Black bean and cheese empanadas

Pulled chicken with cabbage, crema

Chicken tortilla soup

Queso (3-cheese blend)

Ceviche (shrimp)

Ceviche (salmon)

Entrees

Roasted half chicken

Pork carnitas

Tampiquena (beef + enchilada)

Chile relleno (black bean, quinoa, corn, tomato)

Roasted mushroom huarache (spicy sauce)

Red chile chicken

Angus beef NY strip steak

Cocoa-rubbed short ribs

Taco (crispy shrimp)

Taco (beef)

Taco (mushrooms)

Enchiladas (duck)

Enchiladas (beef brisket)

Salmon pipian (vegetable sauté)

Pork shank

Cheeseburger grande

Ribeye steak

Parrilladas (grilled beef, shrimp, chorizo, chicken)

Grilled chorizo

Jumbo shrimp with cilantro

Taco (tuna)

Taco (red chile chicken)

Taco (duck)

Taco (pork)

Enchiladas (roasted chicken)

Enchiladas (roasted mushrooms with cheese)

Sides

Black beans, only if vegetarian

Mexican fried rice

Fried ripe plantains and crème

Mac N Queso

Mexican rice

Black beans and rice (only if vegetarian)

Sweet corn

Frijoles borrachos (bacon, tomato, onion)

Recommendations:

Appetizer: Quesadilla, if vegetarian; or guacamole with pineapple pico de gallo

Salad: Chopped salad, without egg

Entrée: Mushroom taco or black bean/rice (only if vegetarian)

Dessert:

Overall: ☑ 👍 ☐ 👎

Pizza restaurant: Brooklyn, NY

Pizzas

Cheese pizza

Everything pizza (cheese, beef, pepperoni, etc.)

Special pizza (sausage, artichoke hearts)

White pizza

Veggie pizza (cheese, olives, onions, shallots, etc.)

Calzone

Stuffed pizza dough

Nutella calzone

Nothing to choose here.

Recommendations:

   Appetizer:

   Salad:

   Entrée:

   Dessert:

   Overall: ☐ 👍 ☑ 👎

Russian restaurant: Arlington, VA

Appetizers
Blini (crepe like pancakes with beef)

Samsa (rolled butter dough with lamb)

Potato pirozhki (pie with potatoes, onion, sour cream)

Chebureki (deep-fried turnover with beef)

Meat pirozhki (pie with filo dough + beef + crème)

Salads
Tomato salad

Radish and cucumber salad

Vinaigrette salad (potatoes, carrots, onions)

Olivier (Russian potato salad) (eggs, chicken)

Fish under coat (herring with potatoes, carrots)

Soups
Borsch (beets and cabbage, sour cream) (no cream)

Mastava (beef, rice, potatoes, vegetables)

Shurpa (lamb, potatoes, carrots, chickpeas)

Entrees
Manti (Uzbek dumplings with lamb)

Dolma (beef, rice in grape leaves, sour cream)

Lamb shashlyk (lamb, onions, rice)

Kazan kabob (lamb chops)

Beef Stroganoff (beef in sour cream and tomato)

Russian roasted salmon

Lula kabob

Golupsi (cabbage leave with ground beef)

Pelmeni (boiled dumplings with beef, yogurt)

Chicken kiev (fried with steamed vegetables)

Chicken shashlyk (chicken, onions, rice)

Lamb shank

Plov (lamb, rice, carrots, chickpeas, raisins)

Veal chops

Vareniki (ravioli with potato, mushrooms, sour cream)

Sides
French fries

Steamed vegetables

Mashed potatoes

White rice

Recommendations:
- Appetizer:
- Salad: Tomato salad or radish/cucumber salad or vinaigrette salad
- Entrée: Borsch without sour cream or steamed vegetables
- Dessert:
- Overall: ☐ 🔥 ☑ 🌱

Seafood restaurant: Miami Beach, FL

Appetizers
Shrimp cocktail
Conch fritters
Stuffed clams
Snow crab claws

Wild oysters
Fried calamari
Coconut shrimp
Chilled seafood tower

Soups and Salads
Stone crab bisque
Chopped salad (with eggs, cheese)
Caesar salad

Manhattan clam chowder
Cole slaw
Wedge of lettuce

Entrees
Stone crabs
Fried lobster tails
Sea scallops
Lobster mac and cheese
Ginger salmon
Cod
Red snapper
NY strip steak
Fillet mignon
Chopped tenderloin
Fried chicken

King crab legs
Jumbo lump crab cakes
Shrimp
Seafood paella
Blackened mahi
Grouper
Lobster roll
Bone-in ribeye steak
Skirt steak
Classic burger

Sides
Hash browns potatoes
Corn with lime butter
Brussels sprouts
Baked potato
Asparagus, steamed, grilled, or fried

Grilled tomatoes (spinach, cheese)
Creamed spinach
French fries
Skinny fried sweets with cinnamon sugar

Recommendations:
  Appetizer:
  Salad: Wedge of lettuce, but only if you know what is in the salad dressing
  Entrée: Only sides, such as Brussels sprouts or asparagus or baked potato without butter
  Dessert:
  Overall: ☐ 👍 ☑ 👎

Spanish restaurant: New Orleans, LA

Appetizers

Citrus and Vermouth marinated olives

Papas bravas with aioli and piquillo
  pepper puree
Blistered shishito peppers
Grilled Spanish octopus

Charred romaine with roasted vegetables

Mixed roasted mushrooms, crouton,
  egg yolk

Griddled sourdough with boquerones
  and olives
Beef shank and potato bombas with aioli

Gambas al ajillo with oregano and sherry
Beet salad with Spanish blue cheese
  and walnuts
Wilted broccoli with brown butter, capers,
  garlic

Entrees

Lamb and beef albondigas with tomato,
  cheese
Scallops a la plancha with saffron bacon

Braised pork shank with crispy potatoes
Boneless ribeye with onion and salsa
  verde

Seared yellow-fin tuna with olive, lemon,
  oregano
Seared gulf fish a la lancha with green
  romesco
Seafood paella with shrimp, clams, mussels

Recommendations:
  Appetizer:
  Salad:
  Entrée:
  Dessert:
  Overall: ☐ 🔥 ☑ 🌶

Steak House restaurant: Chicago, IL

Appetizers
Shrimp cocktail
Jumbo lump crab cake
Sesame-seared tuna
Florida stone crab claws

Oysters on the half shell
Crabmeat avocado
Alaskan red king crab cocktail

Soups and salads
House salad
Loaded wedge
Caprese salad

Cole slaw
Caesar
Cobb salad

Entrees
Prime rib French dip
Heritage Berkshire pork chop
New York strip steak
T-bone steak
Tomahawk steak
Prime rib steak
Faroe island salmon
Planked Lake Superior whitefish

Gold coast fillet sliders
Baby back ribs
Bone-in strip steak
Porterhouse steak
Marinated skirt steak
Fillet mignon
Miso-marinated Chilean sea bass
Alaskan red king crab legs

Sides
French fries
Mashed potatoes
Creamed spinach
Double-baked potato
Broccoli

Baked potato
Sweet potato
Sautéed mushrooms
Grilled asparagus
Sautéed spinach

Desserts:
Texas pecan pie
Macadamia turtle pie
Crème Brûlée

Carrot cake
Chocolate mousse pie
Ice cream

Recommendations:
   Appetizer:
   Salad:
   Entrée: Only sides
   Dessert:
   Overall: ☐ 👍 ☑ 👎

Thai restaurant: Toronto, Canada

Appetizers

Edamame
Curry puff
Chicken wings
Crispy crab wonton
Fried fish cake
Wonton soup
Chicken tom yom
Green salad (ginger dressing)

Fried Wonton
Fried fish ball
Veggie spring roll, if not fried
Chicken satay
Steam dumpling
Shrimp tom yum
Chicken tom khar
Labb (spicy chicken or pork)

Curry

Red curry
Green curry

Panang curry

Stir-Fried Dishes

Garlic sauce with meat
Mixed vegetable sauce
Cashew nut sauce

Basil sauce with ground meat
Ginger sauce
Eggplant lover

Noodles

Pad Thai, if vegetarian option is available
Lo main (noodles with onions, scallions, cabbage)
Pad Woon Sen (bean noodles with egg, scallions)

Lad nar (noodles with meat)
Pad C-Ew (noodles with veggies)

Drunken noodles (with basix, onions, scallions)

Sides

White rice
Sticky rice
Steamed vegetables
Extra tofu
Extra chicken
Extra beef
Extra squid

Brown rice
Steamed noodles
Extra egg
Extra cashew nut
Extra pork
Extra shrimp
Peanut sauce

Recommendations:
    Appetizer: Edamame
    Salad: Green salad with ginger dressing
    Entrée: Pad Thai, if vegetarian or steamed vegetables with brown rice
    Dessert:
    Overall: ☑ 👍 ☐ 👎

Turkish restaurant: Dallas, TX

Appetizers
Red lentil soup, if vegetarian
Baba ghanoush
Stuffed grape leaves
Eggplant salad
Sheppard salad
White bean salad
Borek (phyllo roll with cheese)
Zucchini pancakes

Hummus
Spinach tarator
Spicy vegetables
Cacik (yogurt with labneh and cucumbers)
Agora salad
Octopus salad
Kibbeh balls (lamb and onions)
Falafel, if not fried

Entrees
Ravioli (lamb)
Baby okra
Chicken kabab
Lamb gyro
Lamb meatballs
Lamb chops
Yogurt chicken adana
Yogurt lamb gyro
Falafel wrap
Chicken shish wrap
Lamb adana wrap
Whole branzino
Swordfish

Hunkar begendi (eggplant puree)
Chicken sauté
Chicken shish
Lamb adana (peppers, rice, cabbage)
Lamb shish
Mixed grill
Yogurt chicken shish
Yogurt lamb meatballs
Chicken adana wrap
Lamb gyro wrap
Lamb meatballs wrap
Salmon

Sides
Feta cheese
Red cabbage
French fries
Plain yogurt
Hot sauce
Calamari sauce

Turkish pide bread
Traditional rice
Sautéed vegetables
White sauce
Tahini sauce

Recommendations:
Appetizer: Baba ghanoush or eggplant salad or humus
Salad: Baby okra
Entrée: Rice with vegetables
Dessert:
Overall: ☑ 🔥 ☐ 🌶

Vegetarian restaurant: New York City, NY

Appetizers

Buffalo Arancini (blue cheese)

Roasted cauliflower

Sweet potato gnocchi

Jackfruit tacos

Caesar salad

10 vegetable stir-fry

Cape Cod cakes

Hand-cut fries

Crispy artichokes (quinoa-flour)

Nachos

Greek salad

Pizza (gluten free)

Entrees

Veggie burger

Tofu BLT

Seitan piccata

Salmon tofu (beet-marinated grilled tofu)

Savory seitan

Southern seitan

Grilled cheese and soup

Lasagna (with tofu)

Curried stuffed sweet potato

Sides

Ginger garlic braised tofu

Brown rice

Sautéed kale

Field greens

Black beans

Brussels sprouts

Broccoli rabe

Mashed potatoes

Desserts

Chocolate ganache

Apple strudel, if vegan

Tiramisu

Cashewtopia ice cream, if vegan

Recommendations:

    Appetizer: Many to choose from

    Salad: Many to choose from

    Entrée: Many to choose from

    Dessert: Many to choose from

    Overall: ☑ 👍👍👍   ☐ 👎

Airport food options: Miami International Airport

Restaurants Inside Terminal
1. Budweiser Brewhouse
2. Burger King
3. Pizza Hut
4. Café La Caretta (Cuban classics)
5. Café Versailles (Cuban classics)
6. Icebox Café
7. Ku-Va (Cuban classics)
8. Spring Chicken (Southern comfort food)
9. Shula's Bar & Grill (steaks)
10. Au Bon Pain
11. 305 Pizza
12. Bacardi Mojito Bar
13. Beaudevin (wine bar)
14. Clover Irish Pub
15. Clubhouse One (burgers)
16. The Counter (burgers)
17. Corona Beach House (burgers)
18. Dunkin Donuts
19. Einstein Bagels
20. Estefan Kitchen Express (Cuban food)
21. Fig & Fennel (Mediterranean-themed sandwiches)
22. Halfmoon Empanadas
23. Islander Bar & Grill (Caribbean food)
24. Kpse Ciervp Teqileria (Mexican food)
25. Juan Valdes Café (coffee and light breakfast)
26. Manchu Wok (Chinese food)
27. Nathan's Famous Hot Dogs
28. Starbucks
29. Sushi Maki
30. TGI Friday's (American food)
31. Villa Pizza
32. Wendy's

Recommendations of healthy places to eat from the above list:
Each airport attracts unique food vendors, some of which have "enlightened" food choices.
Occasionally, you can find healthy options.

Whole Foods buffet

Salads

Cabbage

Broccoli

Spinach

Lettuce

Tomatoes

Other vegetables

Entrees

Chicken Korma (Indian)

Country fried chicken (North Florida)

Tacos con Carne (Mexico)

Chile glazed Thai chicken (Thailand)

Picadillo (Cuban)

Chicken Cacciatore (Italian)

Greek salad

Yucca con Questo

Arroz con Pollo

Recommendations:

Salad: Salad bar

Entrée: Depends upon what is available in the location. Usually, ingredients are listed.

Overall: ☑ 👍 ☐ 👎

Airplane snacks

American Airlines
Biscoff cookies   Pretzels
Love corn

JetBlue Airlines
Cjeez-It   PopCorners
88Acres Seed Bar Thins   Goodie Girl Mini Cookies

Delta Airlines
Cheez-Its   Squirrel Brand Almonds
KIND Dark Chocolate Chunk Bars   Biscoff cookies

Nothing healthy to snack on. Bring your own.

When you are flying internationally or on some flights longer than 3 hours or if you are flying business or first class, you might be provided one or more meals. Every carrier will have vegetarian option, or a vegan option or a fruit plate. Some carriers use meal vendors that are better than others. Don't expect too much and you will be fine.

Fast Food Restaurants

Healthier Choices Are Highlighted in Gray

Arby's

Beer battered fish
Chicken club wrap
Double beef N' cheddar
Roast turkey ranch and bacon sandwich
Spicy prime rib cheesesteak
Loaded Italian
Roast beef
Smokehouse brisket
Chicken club wrap
Jalapeno bacon ranch wrap

Buffalo chicken slider
Classic prime rib cheesesteak
Mozzarella sticks
Smokehouse brisket
Greek gyro
Reuben
Roast beef gyro
Turkey gyro
Creamy Mediterranean chicken wrap
Roast turkey and Swiss

BurgerFi

Double burger
Ultimate bacon cheeseburger
Spicy wagyu
Beef and VegeFi burger with cheese
Vegan beyond burger
Chicken sandwich
Fried chicken tenders
Wagyu hotdog with kraut
French fries
Custard cups

Double burger with cheese
Wagyu, brisket, bacon, cheese
Burger, cheese, egg, hash browns
Beyond burger
VegiFi burger (from quinoa)
Spicy fried chicken sandwich
Wagyu beef hotdog
Wagyu hotdog with cheese and sauce
Onion rings
Milkshakes

Burger King

Whopper
Whopper with cheese and bacon
Double whopper
Impossible whopper
Single-quarter-pound king
Burger with onion rings
Chicken sandwich
Chicken fries
Classic fries
Sundae pie
Vanilla shake

Whopper with cheese
Spicy whopper with cheese
Triple whopper with cheese
Whopper Jr.
Double cheeseburger
Texas double whopper
Spicy chicken sandwich
Chicken nuggets
Onion rings
Oreo cookies shake
Soft serve cup

Chick-fil-A

Chicken sandwich

Spicy chicken sandwich

Grilled chicken club sandwich

Chicken nuggets

Chicken wrap

Spicy Southwest salad

Side salad

Chicken sandwich with cheese

Grilled chicken sandwich

Smokehouse BBQ bacon sandwich

Grilled nuggets

Cobb salad

Market salad

Chipotle Mexican Grill

Burrito bowl

Quesadilla (beef, chicken, or veggies)

Salad

Chips

Chips and guacamole

Burrito

Three tacos

Build your own salad

Chips and salsa

Chips and queso blanco

Church's Chicken

Texas-sized meal (chicken, 2 sides, biscuit)

Two-piece chicken

Jalapeno cheese bombers

French fries

Baked mac and cheese

Jalapeno peppers

Mashed potatoes

Chicken sandwich

Chicken tenders

Corn on the cob

Honey-butter biscuit

Fried okra

Cole slaw

Apple pie

Einstein Brothers

Big breakfast burrito

Jalapeno bacon on a bun

Avocado toast

Jalapeno cheddar on bagel

Power protein bagel

Green chile bagel

Asiago cheese bagel

Chocolate chip bagel

French toast bagel

Plain bagel

Sesame bagel

Honey whole-wheat bagel

Poppy seed bagel

Ancient grain bagel

Cream cheese (plain, onion and chive, veggie)

Turkey, bacon, and avocado on bagel

Turkey and cheddar cheese on bagel

Ham and Swiss on bagel

Plain bagel pepperoni

Chocolate chip cookie

Blueberry muffin

Twice-baked hash browns

Texas Brisket egg sandwich

Jalapeno bacon on bagel

Six cheese bagel

Apple cinnamon bagel

Spinach Florentine bagel

Cheesy hash brown bagel

Blueberry bagel

Cinnamon sugar bagel

Pretzel bagel

Everything bagel

Cinnamon raisin bagel

Cranberry bagel

Onion bagel

Pumpernickel bagel

Cream cheese (jalapeno salsa, strawberry)

Tasty turkey on bagel

Avocadoes veg on bagel

Nova on bagel

Pizza bagel with cheese

Chocolate chip coffee cake

Greek yogurt cherry pastry

Jamba Juice

Electric berry lemonade smoothie

Caribbean passion smoothie

Summer blackberry smoothie

Acai super-antioxidant smoothie
(soymilk, acai)

Orange-C booster smoothie (OJ + sherbet)

Chunky strawberry bowl

Vanilla blue sky bowl

Impossible sausage sandwich

Spring veggie (egg, yogurt whip cream,
cheese)

Turkey sausage wrap

Aloha pineapple smoothie

Go getter (plant based, veggies and fruit)
smoothie

Apple n' greens smoothie

Matcha green tea smoothie (soymilk)

Acai primo bowl

Island pitaya bowl

Oatmeal with soymilk

Classic sausage, egg, cheese

Belgian waffle

Sweet pretzel

Jersey Mike's Subs

Ham and cheese

Veggie

Turkey and provolone

Roast beef and provolone

Provolone, applewood bacon, ham, turkey

Bacon, lettuce tomato

Provolone, ham, salami

Grilled portabella and Swiss cheese

Portobello chicken cheese steak

Chipotle cheese steak

Grilled onions, peppers, American cheese

Onions, peppers, mushrooms, chicken,
cheese

Lettuce, tomato, mayo chicken, cheese

Chips

Brownie

Provolone and ham

Provolone, ham, prosciuttini

Tuna fish

Provolone, ham, prosciuttini, salami

Beef, Swiss cheese, bacon, mayo

Provolone, prosciuttini, cappacualo

Ham, provolone, pepperoni

Portabella cheese steak

Onions peppers, American cheese

Big Kahuna cheese steak

Onions, peppers, cheese, chipotle mayo

Bacon, lettuce, tomato, cheese, ranch
dressing

Hot sauce, lettuce, tomato, cheese,
blue cheese

Cookie

Tastykake

Long John Silvers

Wild Alaska Pollock: sandwich or taco

Shrimp

Fried cod

Fried chicken

Grilled shrimp

Grilled salmon tacos

Coleslaw

Rice

Corn

Chocolate cream pie

Popcorn shrimp

Shrimp and chicken

Fish and chicken

Grilled salmon

Grilled salmon bowl

Grilled shrimp tacos

French fries

Green beans

Hush puppies

Strawberry swirl cheesecake

KFC

Chicken sandwich	Chicken tenders
Max and cheese	French fries
Biscuits	8-piece bucket of chicken
Chicken breast	Chicken drum and thigh
Fried wings	Chicken pot pie
Chicken bowl	French fries
Mashed potatoes and gravy	Cole slaw
Gravy	Corn

McDonald's

Big Mac	Quarter pounder with cheese
Double quarter pounder with cheese	Quarter pounder with cheese deluxe
McDouble	Quarter pounder with cheese and bacon
Cheeseburger	Double cheeseburger
Hamburger	Spicy deluxe crispy chicken sandwich
Crispy chicken sandwich	Spicy crispy chicken sandwich
Deluxe crispy chicken sandwich	Chicken McNuggets
McChicken	Fillet-O-Fish
French fries	Apple slices
Glazed pull apart donut	Apple fritter
Blueberry muffin	Cinnamon roll

Popeye's

Classic flounder fish sandwich	Spicy flounder fish sandwich
Surf and turf	¼ lb. popcorn shrimp meal
Spicy chicken sandwich	Classic chicken sandwich
12-piece chicken family meal	Chicken tenders, 10 pieces
Mac and cheese	Cajun fries
Mashed potatoes with Cajun gravy	Red beans and rice
Coleslaw	Biscuits

Shake Shack

Buffalo chicken	Chicken shack
Avocado bacon chicken	Chicken bites
ShackBurger	SmokeShack
Avocado bacon burger	'Shroom burger (with cheese, wheat, egg, soy)
Cheeseburger	Bacon cheeseburger
Grilled cheese	Hotdog
Buffalo spiced fries	Buffalo spiced cheese fries
French fries	Cheese fries
Bacon cheese fries	Chocolate pie shake
Shakes	Floats

Sonic Drive-In

Cheeseburger
Bacon double cheeseburger
Buffalo sauced jumbo popcorn chicken
Crispy chicken tenders
Classic grilled chicken sandwich
Chili cheese Coney Island hotdog
Footlong quarter-pound Coney
Grilled cheese sandwich
Potato tots
Fries
Ched 'R peppers
Quarter-pound double cheeseburger
Jumbo popcorn chicken
Honey BBQ-sauced jumbo popcorn chicken
Crispy chicken sandwich
Chicken slinger
All-American hotdog
Corndog
Mozzarella sticks
Chili cheese tots
Chili cheese fries
Handmade onion rings

Starbucks

Coffee
Frappuccino
Impossible breakfast sandwich
Double-smoked bacon, cheddar, and egg
    sandwich
Sausage, cheddar, and egg sandwich
Spinach, feta, egg white wrap
Kale and mushroom egg bites
Egg white and roasted red pepper egg
    whites
Ham and Swiss on baguette
Chicken caprese on ciabatta
Tomato and mozzarella on focaccia
Cheese trio protein box
Chickpea bites and avocado protein box
Eggs and cheddar protein box
Cheese and fruit protein box
Dipped Madeleines
Dark chocolate granola
Banana
Squirrel brand—classic almond
Rolled and steel-cut oatmeal and
    blueberries
Berry trio parfait
Tea
Cold drinks
Bacon, gouda, and egg sandwich
Turkey bacon, cheddar, and egg white
    sandwich
Roasted ham, Swiss, and egg sandwich
Avocado spread
Bacon and gruyere egg bites
Crispy grilled cheese on sourdough

Turkey, provolone, and pesto on ciabatta
Chicken and bacon on brioche
Eggs and gouda protein box
Cheddar and uncured salami protein box
Chicken and hummus protein box
PB&J protein box
Vanilla biscotti with almonds
Shortbread cookies
Rip van Waffles—honey and oats
Squirrel brand fruit and nuts
Peter Rabbit organic apple and grape juice
Rolled and steel-cut oatmeal

Strawberry overnight gains

Subway

Sweet onion teriyaki sub
Supreme meats sub
Baja turkey avocado sub
Baja chicken and bacon sub
Black Forest ham sub
Chicken and bacon ranch sub
Italian BMT sub
Oven-roasted turkey sub
Tuna sub
Mozza meat sub
Club sub
Honey mustard rotisserie-style chicken sub
Baja steak and jack sub
Buffalo chicken sub
Cold-cut combo sub
Meatball marinara sub
Roast beef sub
Veggie delight sub

Taco Bell

Cheesy gordita crunch taco	Doritos cheesy gordita crunch taco
Soft taco	Crunchy taco
Steak white hot ranch fry's burrito	White hot ranch fries burrito—veggie
Bean burrito	Beefy 5-layer burrito
Quesarito	Burrito supreme
Crunchwrap supreme	Nacho fries
Nachos BellGrande	Chicken Chipotle melt
Chips and nacho cheese sauce	Cheesy fiesta potatoes
Black bean chalupa supreme	Black bean crunchwrap
Chalupa supreme	Crunchwrap supreme
Power menu bowl	Black bean quesarito
Cinnamon twists	Black beans and rice
Cinnabon delights	

Wendy's

Big bacon cheddar cheeseburger	Big bacon cheddar cheeseburger double
Big bacon cheddar cheeseburger triple	Bourbon bacon cheeseburger
Bourbon bacon cheeseburger double	Dave's single
Dave's double	Dave's triple
Baconator	Son of baconator
Son of baconator	Big bacon classic
Jr. cheeseburger deluxe	Jr. cheeseburger
Double stack	Jr. Hamburger
Hot honey chicken sandwich	Hot honey chicken sandwich (grilled)
Big bacon cheddar chicken	Spicy big bacon cheddar
Grilled big bacon cheddar chicken	Spicy chicken nuggets
Spicy chicken sandwich	Grilled chicken sandwich
Asiago ranch classic chicken club	Spicy Asiago ranch club
Crispy chicken BLT	Spicy chicken
Chicken nuggets	Crispy panko fish sandwich

Casual Dining Restaurants

Healthier Choices Are Highlighted in Gray

Benihana

Appetizers

Edamame

Shrimp/chicken/vegetable tempura

Shrimp sauté

Tokyo wings

Sashimi sampler (tuna, salmon, snapper)

Crispy rice

Chicken rice

Benihana salad

Miso soup

Spicy edamame

Pan-fried gyoza dumpling

Soft shell crab

Tuna poke

Seared tuna

Chili ponzu yellowtail

Spicy chicken rice

Seaweed salad

Benihana onion soup

Entrees

Lotus tempura roll

Alaskan roll

Las Vegas roll (deep fried)

Sumo roll (baked)

Sashimi (tuna, yellowtail, salmon, eel, Krab)

Dragon roll

Spicy tuna roll

Philadelphia roll

Vegetable roll

California roll

Yakisoba (sautéed noodles in veg sauce)

Hibachi Chateaubriand

Teriyaki steak

Hibachi steak

Fillet mignon

Hibachi salmon with avocado sauce

Hibachi scallops

Surf side (shrimp, calamari, scallops)

Hibachi shrimp

Steak and chicken breast

Shrimp lover's roll

Chili shrimp roll

Shrimp crunchy roll

Lobster roll

Sashimi (snapper, smoked salmon, shrimp)

Rainbow roll

Spicy salmon roll

Salmon roll

Cucumber roll

Eel roll

Spicy tofu steak

Hibachi chicken

Spicy hibachi chicken

Teriyaki chicken

Spicy hibachi shrimp

Twin lobster tails

Colossal shrimp

Lobster tail and scallops

Hibachi tuna steak

Fillet mignon and scallops

Desserts

Strawberry mochi

Rainbow sherbet

Edy's ice cream

Green tea ice cream

☑ No healthy options to choose.

Bonefish Grill

Appetizers

Bang shrimp

Tempura crunch sashimi tuna

Crab cakes

Beef and ginger potstickers

Corn chowder and lump crab

Caesar salad (without cheese or
   anchovies)

Ahi tuna poke

Imperial dip (seafood, cheese, chips)

Calamari

Crab fries

House salad (heart of palm, olives,
   tomato, citrus)

Cobb salad

Entrees

Atlantic salmon

Chilean sea bass

Rainbow trout

Bone-in pork chop

Tuna poke bowl cod imperial

Cold water lobster tails

Fillet mignon

Chicken with goat cheese

Pork chop

Crispy fried shrimp

Mahi-mahi

Scallops and shrimp

Chicken breast

Pasta with red sauce

Parmesan-crusted rainbow trot

Half-pound burger

Sirloin steak

Chicken marsala

Fish and chips

Blackened fish tacos

Sides

Steamed asparagus

Seasonal vegetables

Garlic whipped potatoes

Jasmine rice

Desserts

Macadamia nut brownie

Warm cookies

Classic cheesecake

Key lime cake

☑ No healthy options to choose.

Cheesecake Factory

Appetizers

Tossed green salad

Greek salad

Sliders

Quesadilla

Avocado eggrolls

Fried macaroni and cheese

Sweet corn tamale cakes with sour cream

Eggroll sampler

Buffalo wings

Thai lettuce wraps with avocado

Caesar salad (without cheese or anchovies)

Chopped salad with chicken

Chicken pot stickers

Tex-Mex eggrolls with spicy chicken

Pretzel bites with cheddar cheese fondue

Fried chicken sliders

Hot spinach and cheese dip

Fried calamari

Factory nachos with cheese, guacamole, sauce

Thai lettuce wraps with chicken

Entrees

Fish and chips

Shrimp and chicken gumbo

Jamaican black pepper shrimp

Grilled salmon

Carne Asada steak

Hibachi steak

Grilled ribeye steak

Asian chicken salad

Hamburger

Crispy chicken sandwich with ranch dressing

Grilled turkey burger

Chicken pasta

Lemon-garlic shrimp

Steak medallions

Fried shrimp platter

Shrimp scampi

Jamaican black pepper chicken

Miso salmon

Steak Diane

Chargrilled NY steak

Fillet mignon

Mexican tortilla salad

Impossible burger

Crispy chicken sandwich with sriracha mayo

Chicken soft tacos

Tuscan chicken

Grilled salmon

Desserts

Original cheesecake

Pineapple upside-down cheesecake

Low-licious cheesecake

Carrot cake

Tiramisu cake

Fresh strawberry cheesecake

Chocolate caramelicious cheesecake and snickers

Cinnabon cinnamon swirl cheesecake

Warm apple crisp

Fresh strawberry shortcake

☑ No healthy options to choose.

Chuck E. Cheese

Appetizers
Sauced meatballs

Appetizer sampler

Garden salad

Cheesy bread

French fries

Entrees
Build your own pizza

Five meat pizza

Gluten free with cheese pizza

Supreme (pepperoni, sausage, beef, olives, etc.)

Veggie pizza

Chicken wings with various sauces

Desserts
Unicorn churros

Customized cakes

Dippin Dots

☑ No healthy options to choose.

Cracker Barrell

Entrees

Three-cheese squash casserole
Southern fried chicken
Chicken n' dumplings
Chicken potpie
Turkey n' dressing
Pot roast
Grilled sirloin steak
Barrel cheeseburger
Sugar cured ham
Barrel-cut sugar ham
Lemon pepper grilled rainbow trout
Fried cod fillets
Country vegetable plate with biscuits

Country fried steak with sides
Sunday homestyle chicken
Maple bacon grilled chicken
Chicken fried chicken
Roast beef
Meatloaf
Hamburger steak
Cheeseburger with bacon
Country ham
Country fried pork chops
Country fried shrimp
Homestyle chicken BLT
Homestyle chicken salad

Sides

Loaded hashbrown casserole tots

Biscuit beignets

Desserts

Strawberry shortcake

Double chocolate fudge Coca-Cola cake

☑ No healthy options to choose.

Denny's

Appetizers

Loaded jalapeno cheddar tots

Zesty nachos

Smothered cheese fries

Creamy chicken soup

Clear soup

Grilled chicken cobb soup

Chicken tenders

Pancakes puppies

Chicken wings

Creamy mushroom soup

Chicken Caesar salad

Beef bacon cobb salad

Classics (entrees)

Spaghetti Bolognese

Fish and chips

Belgian waffle slam (with 2 eggs, bacon)

Lumberjack slam (with ham)

Grand slam slugger (pancakes, eggs, bacon)

Original buttermilk pancakes

Strawberry citrus pancakes

Banana strawberry chocolate chip pancakes

Philly melt (beef or chicken)

BLT

Grand Slamwich (eggs, sausage bacon)

Ultimate omelet (sausage, bacon, peppers)

Philly cheesesteak omelet

Supreme skillet (sausage, spinach, peppers)

Sweet and tangy chicken skillet

Beef bacon cheeseburger

Chicken beef bacon classic

Spicy mayo burger

Sirloin steak and shrimp

Oxtail fried rice

Chicken porridge

Salmon fillet

Fit slam (egg whites scrambled with spinach)

French toast slam (with eggs, bacon)

All-American slam (with cheese, bacon)

Dulce de leche crunch pancakes

Banana pancakes

Salted caramel and banana cheese pancakes

Ham and egg sandwich

Club sandwich (chicken, ham, bacon)

Super Bird (chicken, ham, cheese)

Loaded veggie omelet (spinach, mushrooms)

Ham and cheese omelet

Crazy spicy skillet (chorizo, jalapeno, mushrooms)

Fit fare veggie skillet (potatoes, broccoli, eggs)

Double cheeseburger

Beef bacon slamburger

Sweet and tangy beef bacon burger

Sirloin steak

Sirloin steak and eggs

Padang fried rice (rice, eggs, chicken stew)

Chicken rice

Sides

Sautéed vegetable blend

Steamed rice

Grilled ham

Sweet corn

☑ No healthy options to choose.

Hard Rock Café

Appetizers

Three-cheese and Roma tomato flatbread

Pepperoni flatbread

Wings

All-American sliders

Bruschetta

Southwest chicken flatbread

Classic nachos with beans and cheese sauce

Boneless wings

Cuban sliders

Bangkok spicy shrimp

Entrees

BBQ bacon cheeseburgers

Double-decker double cheeseburger

Legendary burger (with Applewood bacon)

Country burger (smashed and stacked)

Spicy diablo burger

NY strip steak

Twisted mac, chicken and cheese

Smokehouse BBQ combo

Tupelo chicken tenders

Steak salad

Southwest chicken bowl

Big cheeseburger

Impossible burger with cheese

Moving mountains burger (cheese, onion rings)

Swiss mushroom burger

Cowboy ribeye

Fajitas (chicken, steak, or veggies)

Baby back ribs

Cedar plank salmon

Grilled chicken Caesar salad

Grilled salmon noodle bowl

Desserts

New York cheesecake

Ice cream

Hot fudge brownie

Homemade apple cobbler

Diner-style milkshakes

☑ No healthy options to choose.

Houston's

Appetizers

Chilled jumbo shrimp

Spinach and artichoke dip

Traditional salad (egg, bacon,
    croutons, etc.)

Caesar salad (without cheese
    or anchovies)

Sashimi tuna salad

Thai steak and noodle salad (marinated
    fillet)

House-smoked salmon

Tostones (plantains)

Grilled artichokes

Emerald kale and rotisserie chicken

Grilled chicken salad

Cheeseburger

Entrees

House-made veggie burger
    (without bun, cheese)

Ruby red trout

Rotisserie chicken

Barbecue pork ribs

USDA prime fillet

Cheeseburger

Scottish salmon

Double-cut pork chop

The Hawaiian (ribeye steak with glaze)

French dip au jus

Sides

Roasted bell peppers with French feta

Broccoli with lemon

Creamy coleslaw

French fries

Fully loaded baked potato

Braised red cabbage with goat cheese

Freshly shucked creamed corn

Tabbouleh with lemon vinaigrette

Pomme puree

Maybe Healthy Options to Choose.

IHOP

Appetizers
Chicken and veggie salad

Mozza sticks

Entrees
Spicy poblano omelet

Chicken fajita omelet

Bacon temptation omelet

Big steak omelet

Colorado omelet (bacon, beef, sausage)

Spinach and mushroom omelet classic
    burrito

Country breakfast burrito and bowl

Southwest chicken burrito and bowl

Spicy shredded beef and bowl

Strawberry banana French toast

Buttermilk crispy chicken

All-natural roasted turkey

Belgian waffle combo

Spicy poblano fajita burrito and bowl

New Mexico chicken burrito and bowl

Original French toast

Sirloin steak tips

Grilled tilapia

Cheesy chicken bacon

Belgian waffle

Sides
Crispy breakfast potatoes

Hickory-smoked bacon strips

Slice of ham

Buttered toast

Two eggs

Crispy potato pancakes

Pork sausage links

Seasonal fresh fruit

French fries

☑ No healthy options to choose.

J Alexander

Appetizers

Chicken pasta soup

Mr. Jack's crispy chicken tenders

Fire-gilled artichokes with herb butter

Margherita pizza

BBQ pizza

Alex's salad (bacon, cheese, tomatoes)

Faucon salad (bacon bleu cheese,
   egg, croutons)

Cypress salad (crispy chicken tenders,
   pecans)

Dragon salad (beef, noodles, mango,
   avocado)

Deviled eggs

Mexico City spinach con queso

Smoked salmon dip

Sausage pizza

Wild mushroom pizza

Original Caesar salad

Thai kai salad (greens, chicken, peanuts)

Grilled chicken salad

Asian ahi tuna salad

Entrees

Veggie burger (beets, black beans,
   brown rice)

Bacon Swiss burger

French dip

Crispy chicken sandwich

Fish tacos

Steak 'n' fries

New York strip

Fillet mignon with bearnaise (potatoes,
   peppers)

Slow-roasted prime rib

Grilled salmon

Rotisserie chicken

Rattlesnake tagliatelle (spices, peppers,
   chicken)

Old-fashioned cheeseburger

Double-stack burger

Hyde Park (chicken breast, cheese)

Country club (ham, turkey, cheese, bacon)

Panned fish sandwich

Fillet kabob

Steak Maui (garlic, French fries)

Prime rib sandwich

Ahi tuna fillet

Carolina crab cakes

Crispy chicken platter (fries, Cole slaw)

BBQ baby back ribs

Sides

French fries

Orzo and wild rice

Mashed potatoes

Mac and Cheese

Roasted red peppers

Kale and quinoa

Southern Cole slaw

Seasonal green vegetable

Black beans and rice

Loaded baked potato

Israeli couscous

☑ No healthy options to choose.

Legal Sea Foods

Appetizers

Oysters of the day
Colossal naked shrimp cocktail
Tuna poke
Chilled seafood platter
Lobster bisque
Fish tacos
Stuffies (quahogs, chourico, butter)
Organic mussels
Bang cauliflower and green beans

Cape Cod Littleneck clams
Blackened raw tuna tataki
Smoked salmon avocado toast
New England clam chowder
Crispy calamari
Cod fritters
Crab cakes
Ribs

Entrees

Grey sole
North Atlantic Sea scallops
Mexican Street cod
Moroccan grilled swordfish steak
New England baked haddock
Sole imperial (with crabmeat)
Cioppino (clams, mussels, shrimp,
    calamari, etc.)
Gulf of Maine lobster
Grilled tuna steak
Grilled sea scallops
Grilled rainbow trout
Surf and Turf
Citrus beurre blanc fish

Fish and chips
New England clams
Lemon caper grey sole
Sesame crusted yellow-fin tuna
Scampi
Crab cake, shrimp, scallops
Baked lobster mac and cheese

Grilled organic salmon
Grilled cod
Grilled colossal shrimp
Double R Ranch fillet mignon
Cajun spice fish
Grilled butter fish

Sides

Greek salad
Wedge salad (no cheese or bacon)
Herbed rice pilaf
Sichuan green beans
Butter roasted potatoes
Broccoli au gratin
Street corn (with cheese)

House salad
Coleslaw
Jasmine rice
Steamed broccoli
French fries
Fregola salad (sundried tomato nut pesto)

☑ No healthy options to choose.

LongHorn Steakhouse

Appetizers
Wild West shrimp

Spicy chicken bites

Firecracker chicken wraps

White cheddar stuffed mushrooms

Texas onion

Seasoned steakhouse wings

Entrees
Fillet mignon

Sirloin

Fire-grilled T-bone steak

Churrasco

Sirloin and shrimp

Baby back ribs

Hand-breaded chicken

Salmon

Redrock grilled shrimp

Ribeye sandwich

Farm fresh field greens with crispy chicken

7-pepper sirloin

Ribeye

New York strip

Porterhouse

Chop steak

Fillet and lobster

Grilled lamb chops

Parmesan-crusted chicken

Pork chops

Burger

Grilled chicken and strawberry salad

Farm fresh field greens with grilled salmon

Sides
Side salad

Shrimp and lobster chowder

Loaded potato soup

French onion soup

Desserts
Baker's dozen donut bits

Chocolate stampede

Triple chocolate cheesecake

Strawberries and cream shortcake

Kids
Cheeseburger

Grilled chicken tenders

Kraft macaroni and cheese

Chicken tenders

Kid's sirloin steak

☑ No healthy options to choose.

Olive Garden

Appetizers

Fried mozzarella

Calamari

Lasagna fritter

Toasted ravioli

Homemade soup

Stuffed ziti fritter

Spinach-artichoke dip

Shrimp fritto misto

Breadsticks

House salad

Entrees

Chicken alfredo

Chicken parmigiana

Shrimp alfredo

Fettuccine alfredo

Shrimp scampi

Five cheese ziti *al forno*

Cheese ravioli

Chicken scampi

Grilled chicken margherita

6 oz. sirloin steak

Chicken and shrimp carbonara

Tour of Italy

Lasagna classico

Asiago tortellini alfredo with grilled chicken

Seafood alfredo

Chicken marsala

Giant cheese stuffed shells

Eggplant parmigiana

Herb-grilled salmon

Desserts

Black tie mousse cake

Strawberry cream cake

Warm Italian donuts

Tiramisu

Chocolate brownie lasagna

Sicilian cheesecake with strawberry topping

☑ No healthy options to choose.

Outback Steakhouse

Appetizers

Bloomin' onion

Cheese fries

Chicken wings

Grilled shrimp on the barbie

Sydney 'shrooms (battered and fried)

Potato soup

French onion soup

Blue cheese pecan chopped salad

Twisted ribs

Seared peppered ahi

Coconut shrimp

Steakhouse mac and cheese bites

Three-cheese steak dip

Tasmanian chili (all steak; no beans)

Side salad

Entrees

Fillet mignon

Ribeye

Primary rib with creamy sauce

Bone-in NY strip

Gold Coast coconut shrimp

Steamed lobster tail

Bloomin' fried chicken

Drover's ribs and chicken platter

Queensland chicken and shrimp pasta

Grilled chicken on the barbie

Lobster tails

Fried chicken sandwich

Chook o' mine sandwich (cheese, bacon, sauce)

Prime rib sandwich

Brisbane Caesar salad

Center-cut sirloin

Prime rib

Bone-in ribeye

Melbourne porterhouse

Grilled shrimp

Seasoned shrimp

Caramel mustard glazed pork chops

Hand-breaded chicken tenders

Alice Springs chicken (mushrooms, crisp bacon)

Toowoomba salmon

Perfectly grilled salmon

Outbacker burger

Bloomin' burger

Aussie cobb salad

Steakhouse salad

Sides

Homestyle mashed potatoes

Baked potato

Fixed mixed veggies

Seasoned rice

Creamed spinach

Fries

Sweet potato

Fresh seasonal veggies

Steakhouse mac and cheese

Asparagus

☑ No healthy options to choose.

PF Chang China Bistro

Appetizers

Chicken lettuce wraps
BBQ spareribs
Crispy green beans
Tempura calamari
Kung Pao Brussels sprouts
Shishito peppers
Handmade shrimp dumplings
Pork egg rolls
Mandarin crunch salad
Wonton soup
Hot and sour soup
California roll sushi
Spicy tuna roll

Vegetarian lettuce wraps
Northern-style pork spareribs
Edamame
Chili-garlic green beans
Dynamite shrimp
Handmade port dumplings
Vegetable spring rolls
Hand-folded crab wontons
Asian Caesar salad
Egg drop soup
Dynamite roll sushi
Kung Pao dragon roll sushi
Shrimp tempura roll

Entrees

Fire-braised short ribs
Mongolian beef
Crispy honey shrimp
Salt and pepper prawns
Sweet and sour chicken
Ma Po Tofu
Beef with broccoli
Shrimp with lobster sauce
Miso glazed salmon
King Pao chicken
Oolong Chilean Sea bass
Singapore street noodles
Korean glass noodles
GF chicken lettuce wraps
GF Chang's spicy chicken
GF ginger chicken with broccoli
GF beef with broccoli
GF Singapore Street noodles

Chang's spicy chicken
Crispy honey chicken
Peking duck
Pepper steam
Stir-fried eggplant
Buddha's feast, stir-fried
Sesame chicken
Ginger chicken with broccoli
Orange chicken
King Pao shrimp
Pad Thai
Signature lo mein
Fried rice, short rib fried rice
GF egg drop soup
GF Mongolian beef
GF shrimp with lobster sauce
GF fried rice
GF chicken Pad Thai

Maybe Healthy Options to Choose.

Red Lobster

Appetizers

Bacon-wrapped sea scallops
Signature jumbo shrimp cocktail
Langoustine lobster artichoke-and-
    seafood dip
White wine and roasted garlic mussels

Lobster and langoustine pizza
Parrot Isle jumbo coconut shrimp appetizer
Crab-stuffed shrimp Rangoon

Seafood-stuffed mushrooms

Entrees

Salmon, lobster, scallops
Shrimp and shrimp linguini alfredo
Shrimp, scallops, flounder
Lobster, shrimp, salmon
Atlantic salmon
Lobster-topped stuffed flounder
Jumbo coconut shrimp
Snow crab legs
Sirloin
Fillet mignon
Kung Pao noodles with chicken
Cajun chicken linguini alfredo

Fillet mignon and lobster
Lobster
Lobster, scallops, shrimp
Salmon and shrimp
Rainbow trout
Breaded and fried shrimp
Fish and chips
Live Maine lobster
NY strip
Kung Pao noodles with lobster
Shrimp linguine alfredo
Crab linguini alfredo

Sides

New England clam chowder
Bacon mac and cheese
Rice
Baked potato
Mashed potato
Sea-salted French fries
Caesar salad
Half-dozen cheddar bay biscuits

Lobster bisque
Broccoli
Crispy Brussels sprouts
Creamy lobster baked potato
Creamy lobster mashed potato
Coleslaw
House salad

Desserts

Vanilla bean cheesecake
Brownie overboard

Chocolate wave

☑ No healthy options to choose.

Seasons 52

Appetizers

Slow-roasted meatballs

Grilled artichokes with preserved lemon hummus

Ahi tuna tartare

Potato leek soup

Spinach and strawberry salad

Field greens salad

Lump crab cake

Avocado toast

Asparagus soup

Lobster bisque

Romaine Caesar salad (without cheese)

Entrees

Sesame-grilled salmon salad

Maui tuna crunch salad

Rotisserie half chicken

Wood-grilled dry-rubbed pork chop

Brick-oven vegetable gnocchi

Caramelized grilled sea scallops

Fillet mignon and Maine lobster tail

Wood-grilled Kona crusted lamb loin

BBQ chicken salad

Wood-grilled tenderloin salad

Wood-grilled shrimp and grits

Wood-grilled boneless rainbow trout

Wood-grilled fillet mignon

Brick oven–roasted Chilean sea bass

Cedar plank-roasted salmon

Sides

Sweet potato skillet

Crab polenta

Mac "n" cheese

Truffled risotto

☑ No healthy options to choose.

Sizzler

Entrees (only)

Sirloin steak

Cilantro lime barramundi

Shrimp skewers

Double Malibu chicken

Mega bacon burger

Grilled chicken club

Jumbo crispy shrimp

Ribeye steak

Shrimp

Fish n' chips

Dozen chicken wings

Classic burger

Italian herb chicken

☑ No healthy options to choose.

TGI Fridays

Appetizers
Mozzarella sticks
Loaded Southwest potato twists
Whiskey-glazed sample
Wings roulette platter
Green bean fries
Chips and salsa
Philly cheesesteak egg rolls

Spinach and artichoke dip
Amazing blazing pound of cheese fries
Loaded potato skins
Whiskey-glazed sesame chicken strips
Pan-seared pot stickers
Warm pretzels

Entrees
Bucket of bones
Crispy chicken fingers
Sizzling chicken and cheese
Whiskey-glazed burger
Philly cheesesteak burger
Bacon cheeseburger
Cajun shrimp and chicken pasta
Chicken parmesan pasta
Sizzling chicken and shrimp
Simply grilled salmon
Crispy whiskey combo
Bacon ranch chicken sandwich

Whiskey-glazed flat iron steak
Boneless wings
Traditional wings
Loaded cheese fry burger
Beyond Meat cheeseburger
Cheeseburger
Chicken and broccoli alfredo tortellini
Fried shrimp
Fish and chips
Dragon-glazed salmon
Whiskey-glazed chicken sandwich
Southern fried chicken sandwich

Sides and soups
White cheddar broccoli soup
Cheddar mac and cheese
Lemon-butter broccoli
Mashed potatoes
Jasmine rice

Fried shrimp
Coleslaw
Lemon-butter broccoli and cheese
Loaded mashed potatoes
Basket of breadsticks

Desserts
Oreo madness
Brownie obsession

Rainbow cake
Cinnabon caramel pecan cheesecake

☑ No healthy options to choose.

7-Eleven

Sprinkled donuts

Pizza

BBQ bacon cheeseburger

Chicken sandwich

Mini tacos

Spicy garlic chicken roller

Chicken Caesar pasta salad

Chicken salad sandwich

Tuna salad sandwich

Maple flavored sausage, eggs and
   cheese taquitos

Wings

Hotdogs

Black bean burger

Chicken strips

Nachos

Sub sandwich

Chicken Caesar salad

Egg salad sandwich

Pepperoni pasta salad

Spicy empanadas

WaWa

Hoagie sandwiches

Club sandwiches

Brisket sandwiches

Quesadillas

Burritos

Soups (broccoli cheddar, chicken noodle)

Stacked sandwiches

Deli sandwiches

Paninis

Roasted chicken

Chalupas

☑ No healthy options to choose.

Brian's Choices of Healthy Casual Dining Restaurants

None of these restaurants are recommended by us.

If you chose to go to any of them to be with your friends, consider ordering what we have suggested.

It is disappointing to us that these types of casual dining restaurants do not offer any truly healthy food for their customers.

Summary of Suggestions

The National Institute of Aging, a branch of the U.S. Department of Health and Human Services, summarizes what you should do to increase your longevity, maintain cognitive health, and perhaps reduce your chances of developing dementia (www.nia.nih.gov). We have expressed our own recommendations in a chart similar to the way they do. We have added suggestions based on published research and our personal observations.

Suggestions for Longevity

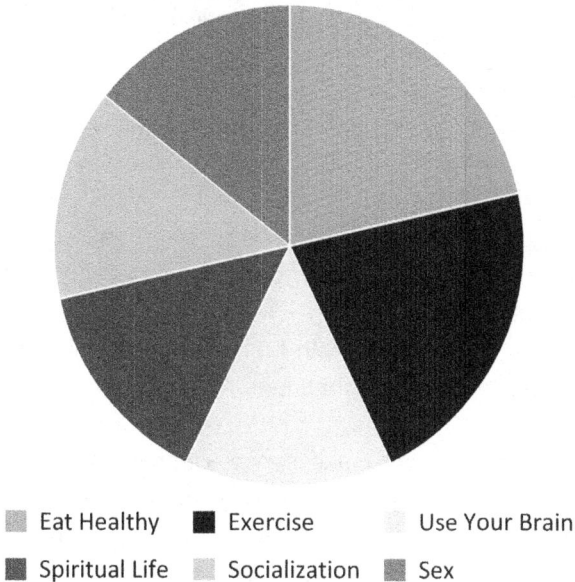

Eat Healthy   Exercise   Use Your Brain
Spiritual Life   Socialization   Sex

We tend to overemphasize eating healthy and doing regular intensive exercise. We know that certain diseases can be prevented, and maybe even reversed, with a plant-based diet. These include type 2 diabetes, arteriosclerotic heart disease, degenerative arthritis, and possibly some types of cancer. Regular, intense exercise has been shown to help patients with type 2 diabetes, arteriosclerotic heart disease, early dementia, early

Parkinson's disease, and probably every person. You should consider the other suggestions in this book and incorporate them into your lives the best you can. Remember, long life is all about making good decisions. Each day should provide you with choices to optimize the chance of a long life.

1. Eat healthy, preferably a plant-based diet, eating organic fruits and vegetables whenever possible.
2. Exercise as recommended by the CDC, unless you are a newbie to exercise, then work your way up to their recommendations. Don't start intensive exercise until you have been cleared by your health care provider.
3. Keep working as long as possible. **When you do retire from work, don't retire from life**. Keep your mind busy, volunteer doing things to help others, read, do crafts, use (or learn to use) the computer, and keep learning new things.
4. Have a spiritual life and have faith in your higher power.
5. Have as many friends and attend as many social events as you can. Loneliness is a hard emotion to deal with. It is important to share your life with your family and friends.
6. Keep having sex.
7. Be careful when going out to dinner. Restaurants are not always friendly places to find healthy food. Have a say in the place you choose to dine.
8. Retire only when you are forced to or when you are sure you have enough money to live on, and you have something productive to do with your newly found time.
9. Be aware of your options with health insurance. The cost of health care is astronomical and continues to rise. Find a good health care provider and stick with them.
10. Keep doing things that make sense: wear a seat belt in a car, use sunscreen when you go outdoors, wear a helmet when you ride your bike even in the neighborhood. Get enough sleep, drink enough water, don't drink and drive, stay away from sugary drinks, wear a hat and sunglasses in the sun, avoid unnecessary medications, socialize with interesting people. Do something meaningful or productive each day, have as many positive thoughts as you can, learn how to manage (or avoid) stress, take time off to be with yourself and your friends, drink as little alcohol as possible, get fresh outdoor air every day, floss your teeth and see your dentist regularly, don't smoke cigarettes, take a nap when you need one.

11. Keep reading about longevity-promoting interventions. The field is wide open; good research is being done. Don't fall for promises from for-profit clinics that seem to "know it all." We don't have all the answers yet. Maybe someday stem cells and other biological factors, not even known to us today, will indeed become the Fountain of Youth that will allow all of us to reach the age of 120.

12. Keep your mind open and be prepared to change when necessary. Remember, there is no one out there who cares about you more than you should care about yourself.

Too Good to Be True

It is part of human nature for some of us to "take the easy way out." Why work hard at something when you can ask someone to do it for you, or you can pay someone to help you? For reasons that are not always clear to us, taking care of your own personal health seems to fall into that area. Could this concept also apply to efforts to increase your longevity?

How many of us know we don't eat healthy yet are unwilling to make a change in what we eat, sometimes even after surviving a life-threatening situation? How many of us are overweight and know we should do something about that, yet are reluctant to get started? How many of us consume too much alcohol, yet always can come up with excuses why we don't have to change? How many of us know we should exercise more, or even start to exercise, yet literally "won't take that first step"? How many of us want to live a long, productive life, yet are paralyzed in starting?

Many people gravitate toward finding the easy way out. People would rather take a pill or injection to lose weight or even undergo a major operation before going to a residential program to get started on a healthy eating program. People would rather book a cruise than stay at a health resort or wellness center for three weeks. People would rather not get started on an exercise program for a variety of reasons, from not liking the way they look in gym clothes to not having a partner to work out with. People would rather not try to learn something new, even if they have the time to do so, especially if it involves the computer. People would rather "close the factory" on sexual relations rather than learning new ways "to do it."

This concept has even spread to longevity. We came across an advertisement in a newspaper for a longevity center located in an exclusive resort community, obviously where wealthy people hang out. Similar ads to this could be found in newspapers, magazines, direct mail, or Internet searches all over. The ad looks something like this.

Anti-Aging Therapy

Regenerative Joint Therapy
Hormone Therapy including using Human Growth Hormone
iv Vitamin Infusions
Year Long Comprehensive Hormone Program
Quarterly Virtual Follow Ups
Call NOW for a FREE consultation

We thought we should explore this claim to see if we should all go there for help. Also, does this (or does any similar center) have any data to share with us on their successes?

A visit to the website of the clinic was a place to start. This center claimed to offer regenerative medicine therapy, hormone replacement, vitamin therapy, skincare, peptide treatments, and PRP injection therapies to help patients gain control over their health and enjoy a better quality of life. We asked ourselves, what does all that mean? Is there any validity to their claims? Can any of those components be done by yourself, or does the clinic have to do it for you? How much does it cost?

What is "Regenerative Medicine"?

According to Wikipedia (https://en.wikipedia.org/wiki/Regenerative_medicine), regenerative medicine deals with the "process of replacing, engineering or regenerating human or animal cells, tissues or organs to restore or establish normal function. This field holds the promise of engineering damaged tissues and organs by stimulating the body's own repair mechanisms to functionally heal previously irreparable tissues or organs. This field also includes the possibility of growing tissues and organs in the laboratory and implanting them when the body cannot heal itself. When the cell source for a regenerated organ is derived from the patient's own tissue or cells, the challenge of organ transplant rejection via immunological mismatch is circumvented."

"Some of the biomedical approaches within the field of regenerative medicine may involve the use of stem cells. Examples include the injection of stem cells or progenitor cells obtained through directed differentiation (cell therapies); the induction of regeneration by biologically active molecules administered alone or as a secretion by infused cells (immunomodulation therapy); and transplantation of in vitro grown organs and tissues (tissue engineering)."

Some major medical centers and research facilities all over the world are actively exploring many different concepts within this space. WebMD (https://www.webmd.com/a-to-z-guides/what-is-regenerative-medicine) tells us that the goal of regenerative medicine is to replace or reboot tissues or organs damaged because of disease, injury, age, or other issues instead of treating symptoms with medication and procedures. Repair can be done at molecular, cellular, or tissue levels. Some of the areas where these concepts are being explored include:

- Type 1 diabetes
- Cardiovascular tissue repair
- Brain injury tissue repair
- Immune system improvement
- Cell therapy
- Tissue engineering
- Skin wounds
- Certain cancers
- Organ transplants

This is an exciting field with an unlimited future. However, perhaps all these conditions should be treated by health care workers in an academic center where they have the best support, best research facilities, and tabulate and even publish their results.

The clinic that we visited claims to treat arthritis, age-related conditions, injuries, and so much more by helping create muscle, bone, and cartilage. They claim their treatments reduce or eliminate joint pain and fight inflammation and disease by promoting new tissue growth that cushions bone and improves movement and function for damaged joints suffering from significant cartilage reduction. This healing reduces pain, inflammation, and other symptoms.

What specific treatments do they offer?
- Hormone replacement treatment for both women and men
- Platelet-rich plasma injections (PRP injections) for wound healing, joint injuries, baldness, promoting healthier-looking skin, and more
- PRP procedures that penetrate the skin's surface and work to jumpstart healthier skin

- Age management
  - Complete history and physical exam
  - Full blood work and diagnostic review
  - Disease risk-management review
  - Hormonal optimization plan
  - Develop and individualized diet and exercise program
- Peptide therapy which promotes healthy cellular function as you age and slow down aging-related symptoms (no specific molecules were listed on their webpage)
- Intravenous vitamin therapy to ensure 100% absorption and achieve rapid results
- Hair restoration, using a nonsurgical approach

We also believe in the appropriate use of hormone replacement therapy, which is discussed in Chapter 6 of this book. We do not believe it should be used for every person and should be prescribed by a physician knowledge-able in this field.

PRP injections are very controversial. PRP injections supposedly work by facilitating the healing process, particularly for injuries that are slow to heal and even chronic. Many astounding claims are being made for this bold new therapy, but through research and consultation with health care providers, it may be possible to figure out if PRP is the right treatment option for you. Platelet-rich plasma is a preparation of the patient's own blood so that it has an above-average concentration of platelets. When injected back into the patient at an injury site, it jump-starts the healing process there. Platelets are tiny, disk-shaped cells in the bloodstream. They serve as the body's fixers, forming blood clots when there is an injury. When an injury activates them, platelets go to work, form blood clots, and rapidly release growth factor proteins to start the healing process. These proteins signal cells in the injured area to grow, differentiate, produce new blood vessels, and lay down fibrous tissue to repair the damage.

PRP therapy involves drawing blood from the patient and separating the red blood cells and most of the white blood cells from the blood plasma and platelets. The platelet-rich plasma contains a highly concentrated amount of these platelets, which are then injected into an injured part of the body. Some centers that perform this procedure will activate the platelets before injection, meaning the clotting process is artificially started before the plate-lets are introduced to the injured area. Some physicians, however, believe it is better to let the platelets activate within the body. When activated, the platelets immediately start to clot and produce growth factor hormones that start healing the affected area.

The body heals itself quickly for most injuries and doesn't require special interventions. PRP treatment is most often used to treat conditions where the healing process is frustratingly slow, such as injuries to the muscles, tendons, or bones. These slow-healing injuries can take months or even years to resolve, but platelet-rich plasma therapy might be able to speed up the process. Most patients will encounter platelet-rich plasma therapy as an elective procedure for sports injuries, chronic tendon injuries, and hip or knee osteoarthritis.

But does it work? The FDA has not approved PRP treatment. The FDA has "cleared" the centrifuges, but not the treatments, so every PRP treatment is technically "off-label" and not covered by insurance. In addition, not all doctors and research scientists agree on which conditions should be treated by PRP. Additionally, there's little consensus on PRP treatment protocols. There are fundamental disagreements about platelet-rich plasma preparation. How many platelets are needed? Should white blood cells be included? What about fibrin, a protein critical to blood clotting? Should it be included? Is activating the platelets before the injection an innovative idea? The answers to all these questions are still being discussed and debated in the medical and scientific community.

According to the website, www.singlecare.com/blog/prp-injection/, here is a list of conditions for which PRP therapy has been used:

- Orthopedists and sports medicine physicians use it for bone, tendon, joint, ligament, and muscle injuries.
- Dentists use PRP injections for tooth extractions, implants, or periodontal surgery to speed up recovery as well as heal soft tissue damage and bones.
- Surgeons use PRP to speed up wound healing and reduce infection rates.
- Plastic surgeons have long used PRP to speed up the healing process of cosmetic surgery, but some use PRP injections to promote connective tissue growth in the face to smooth out wrinkles and restore skin color.
- Dermatologists use PRP along with the medications minoxidil or finasteride to reverse hair loss in men and women. Platelet growth factors stimulate the hair follicles to grow, and the medications manage the effects of testosterone on the hair follicle.

- Some ophthalmologists have started using PRP eye drops directly on the eye surface for corneal ulcers or dry eye injuries. PRP eye drops placed directly on the tear glands can increase tear production.
- Otolaryngologists have used PRP injections to treat hearing or smell loss.
- Finally, some urologists give PRP injections to treat erectile dysfunction.

In the case of the clinic that advertised in the newspaper, it is not clear if the emphasis on the treatment is PRP as the primary therapy for degenerative arthritis versus our program which suggests a plant-based diet (with no animal products) and an intensive exercise program up to tolerance.

As for the use of PRP in the treatment of skin conditions, the American Academy of Dermatology Association on their website, https://www.aad.org/public/cosmetic/younger-looking/platelet-rich-plasma-secret-to-younger-skin, summarizes the information by stating that this is a procedure with little evidence to back it up. While the results are unpredictable, dermatologists are finding that people want to know whether PRP can give them younger-looking skin. They recommend that if you're thinking about trying PRP, see a board-certified dermatologist. These doctors perform more cosmetic procedures than any other type of medical doctor. They have the in-depth training required to evaluate your skin and tell you what proven treatments can be most effective for you. If you and your dermatologist decide that PRP is worth trying, it's important to keep in mind that this is still an unproven treatment. You will be helping to answer the questions that dermatologists still have about this procedure. If you are leaning in that direction, it seems reasonable that you go to a dermatologist with experience in this area.

Their next component is Age Management.

- Complete history and physical exam
- Full blood work and diagnostic review
- Disease risk-management review
- Hormonal optimization plan
- Develop an individualized diet and exercise program

All of that seems routine for any physician who is about to take on a new patient. We do not feel that their emphasis is like ours. We promote diet and exercise above everything else, certainly before we would offer any invasive treatment.

Peptide therapy is something relatively new. This can be classified into two broad categories: well-being/aging and tissue repair. Some of the many peptides that have been used include the following:

Growth hormone
- Growth hormone–releasing peptide (GHRP)
  - **Ipamorelin** (best starting peptide) and **GHRP2** or **GHRP6** (*aka,* ghrelin)
- Growth hormone–releasing hormone (GHRH)
  - **CJC 1295, Sermorelin**

Tissue healing and repair
- **Thymosin B4 (TB4)** is good for tissue healing/repair
- **Body protecting complex aka BPC-157**

Gut Healing—BPC-157 used for gastrointestinal healing.

Immunity, autoimmunity, and tissue healing/repair peptides
- **Thymosin A1(** aka Zadaxin) best for autoimmunity and tissue healing
- **Thymosin B4 (aka TB4) can enhance Thymosin A1**

According to the International Peptide Society, the "majority of naturally occurring peptides bind to cell surface receptors triggering intracellular responses. With over 7,000 peptides that occur naturally in the body, this represents a wide pool of peptides and functions to work with. Naturally occurring peptides have many distinct functions from hormones, growth factors, neurotransmitters and more. Therefore, the use of peptides as therapeutics provides a method of targeting a wide range of cells and manipulating their response."

Despite all the hype, the ongoing clinical trials, and all of these anti-aging clinics popping up all over, there is still a lack of objective scientific data. Bartke (2019) showed that the results of the use of HGH obtained thus far have been disappointing with few documented benefits and many troublesome side effects. Vitale *et al.* (2019) reviewed the use of IGF-1 and longevity and suggested that there may be future clinical applications in promoting healthy aging with optimism, but no large-scale studies are available.

Intravenous vitamin (IV) therapy is another popular procedure that has been claimed to be effective. According to the website of Cedars-Sinai Medical Center (https://www.cedars-sinai.org/blog/iv-vitamin-therapy.html),

IV vitamin therapy is a quick way to provide hydration, but the claim that it bypasses the stomach and goes straight into the bloodstream may not be advantageous. Bypassing your body's built-in safeguards and filters may be harmful. Their conclusion was that IV vitamin therapy is safe, but not any more effective. Houston Methodist's website (https://www.houstonmethodist.org/blog/articles/2021/may/do-iv-hydration-therapy-and-iv-vitamin-therapy-really-work/) also states the same results.

The idea behind both IV hydration therapy and IV vitamin therapy is that delivering specially formulated cocktails of nutrients, vitamins, electrolytes, antioxidants, and sometimes even medications via an IV can help replenish, restore, and detoxify your body quicker than, say, drinking water, eating healthy, or taking a medication orally. "While it's true that an IV can speed up how quickly things enter your bloodstream, it's unlikely that boutique IV therapy companies can actually achieve what they claim—whether that's curing a hangover, boosting your immune system, enhancing focus and the list goes on," explains Dr. Joshua Septimus, Associate Professor of Clinical Medicine and Medical Director of Houston Methodist Primary Care Group Same Day Clinics. Dr. Septimus stresses that these drips are not FDA-approved, meaning there's no clinically validated study confirming that IV hydration therapy and/or IV vitamin therapy have any real benefit to you.

The last piece of information is the cost. Cost varies from center to center. Expect the initial visit to cost between $3,000 and $10,000 depending upon what is ordered. If an expensive treatment plan is initiated, expect another $2,000 for each treatment.

With all this information at your disposal, are you looking for a "quick fix" as a way to avoid having to work hard to follow the suggestions we have recommended?

We feel that diet, exercise, mental stimulation, and socialization are still the key factors to increase longevity. Don't try to replace those by a supplement, an injection, an IV infusion, or an unproved therapy. Work hard on yourself before you look elsewhere, especially if your options of these complementary treatments may not have been adequately researched or studied.

If something sounds too good to be true, it usually is.

APPENDIX D

References

Prologue

The New England Centenarian Study. https://www.bumc.bu.edu/centenarian/

Chapter 1: Healthy Eating

Aung T, Halsey J, Kromhouf D, Gerstein HC, Marchioli R, Tavazzi L, Geleijnse JM, Rauch B, Ness A, Galan P, Chew EY, Bosch J, Collins R, Lewington S, Armitage J, & Clarke R (2018), Associations of omega-3 fatty acid supplement use with cardiovascular disease risk: meta-analysis of 10 trials involving 77,917 individuals. *JAMA Cardiol*, 3:225–233.

Buckner SL, Loprinzi PD, & Loenneke JP (2016), Why don't more people eat breakfast? A biological perspective. *Am J Clin Nutr*, 103:1555–1556.

Campbell TM, & Campbell TC (2006), *The China Study: The Most Comprehensive Study of Nutrition Ever Conducted and the Startling Implications for Diet, Weight Loss, and Long-Term Health*. BenBella Books.

Campisi J, Kapahi P, Lithgow GJ, Melov S, Newman JC, & Verdin E (July, 2019), From discoveries in ageing research to therapeutics for healthy ageing. *Nature*, 571:183–192.

Chousalkar K (2017), *Achieving Sustainable Production of Eggs*, Vol 1. Burleigh Dodds Science Publishing.

D'Auria E, Peroni DG, Sartorio MU, Verduci E, Zuccotti GV, & Venter C (2020), The role of diet diversity and diet indices on allergy outcomes. *Front Pediatr*, 8:545.

DeBoer MD, Agard HE, & Scjarf RO (2015), Milk intake, height & body mass index in preschool children. *Arch Dis Child*, 100:460–465.

DeSoto L (2022), Is breakfast really the most important meal of the day? *MedicalNewsToday*, https://www.medicalnewstoday.com/articles/is-breakfast-really-the-most-important-meal-of-the-day

Eleftheriou D, Benetou V, Trichopoulou A, La Vecchia C, & Bamia C (2018), Mediterranean diet and its components in relation to all-cause mortality: meta-analysis. *Br J Nutr*, 120(10):1081–1097.

Ge L, Sadeghirad B, Ball GDC, da Costa BR, Hitchcock CL, Svendrovski A, Kiflen R, Quadri K, Svendrovski A, Kiflen R, Quadri K, Kwon HY, Karamourian M, Adams-Webber T, Ahmed W, Damanhoury S, Zeraatkar D, Nikkolakipoulou A, Tsuyuki RT, Tian J, Yang K, Guyatt GH, & Johnston BC (2020), Comparison of dietary macronutrient patterns of 14 popular named dietary programs for weight and cardiovascular risk factor reduction in adults: systematic review and network meta-analysis of randomized trials. *BMJ*, 10:369–370.

Hamblin J (2019), The actual reason meat Is not healthy. *The Atlantic*, https://www.theatlantic.com/health/archive/2019/10/meat-wars/599728/

Holt-Lunstat J, Smith TB, Baaker M, Baker M, Harris T, & Stephenson D (2015), Loneliness and social isolation as risk factors for mortality, a meta-analysis. *Prospect Psychol Sci*, 10:227–237.

Lasheras C, Fernandez S, & Patterson AM (2000), Mediterranean diet and age with respect to overall survival in institutionalized, nonsmoking elderly people. *Am J Clin Nutr*, 71:987–992.

Lombardi M, Carbone S, Del Buono MG, ChiabrandoJ G, Vescovo GM, Camilli M, Montone RA, Vergallo R, Abbate A, Biondi-Zoccai, Dixon DL, & Crea F (2021), Omega-3 fatty acids supplementation and risk of atrial fibrillation: an updated meta-analysis of randomized controlled studies. *Eur Heart J*, 10:1093.

Martinez del Campo A, Hamer HA, Marks JA, Turnbaugh PJ, & Baiskus EP (2015), Characterization and detection of a widely distributed gene cluster that predicts anaerobic choline utilization by human gut bacteria. *mBio*, 6:e00042–15.

McCarty MF, DiNicolantonio JJ, Lavie CJ, & O'Keefe JH (2014), Omega-3 and prostate cancer: examining the pertinent evidence. *Mayo Clin Proc*, 89:444–450.

Michaelsson K, Wolk A, Langenskiold S, Basus L, Learning EW, Melhus H, & Byberg L (2014), Milk intake and risk of mortality and fractures in women and men: cohort studies. *BMJ*, 349:1–15.

New England Centenarian Study. bumc.bu.edu/centanarian

Powis S (2019), Fad diets are at best ineffective and can be harmful. *BMJ*, 367:l7083.

Public Health Reports (2015), U.S. Public Health Service recommendation for fluoride concentration in drinking water for the prevention of dental caries. *Public Health Rep*, 130:318–331. https://journals.sagepub.com/doi/abs/10.1177/003335491513000408

Ramadas A, Tham SM, Lalani SA, & Shyam S (2021), Diet quality of Malaysians across lifespan: a scoping review of evidence in a multi-ethnic population. *Nutrients*, 13(4):1380.

Rashwan AK, Asmond AI, Abdelshafy AM, Mo J & Chen W (2023), Plant-based proteins: advanced extraction technologies, interactions, physicochemical and functional properties, food and related applications, and health benefits. *Critical Rev Food Sci Nutr*, https://doi.org/10.1080/10408398.2023.2279696

Rosell MS, Lloyd-Wright Z, Appleby PN, Sanders TAB, Allen NE, & Key TJ (2005), Long-chain n-3 polyunsaturated fatty acids in plasma in British meat-eating, vegetarian, and vegan men. *Am J Clin Nutr*, 82:327–334.

Sinclair D (2019), *Lifespan: why we age and why we don't have to*. Atria Books, New York.

Tucker KL, Morita K, Qiao N, Hannan MT, Cupples A, & Kiel DP (2006), Colas, but not other carbonated beverages, are associated with low bone mineral density in older women: the Framingham study. *Am J Clin Nutr*, 84:836–942.

Wilkinson MJ, Manoogian ENC, & Zadourian A (2020), Ten-hour time-restricted eating reduces weight, blood pressure, and atherogenic lipids in patients with metabolic syndrome. *Cell Metab*, 31:92–104.

Yang Q, Zhang Z, Gregg EW, Glanders WD, Merritt R, & Hu FB (2014), Added sugar intake and cardiovascular diseases mortality among US adults. *JAMA Intern Med*, 10:101.

Zhi-hui L, Xu L, Dai R, Li L, & Wang HJ (2021), Effects of regular breakfast habits on metabolic and cardiovascular disease. *Medicine (Baltimore)*, 100:1–12.

Chapter 2: Exercise

Caliebe A, Kelindorp R, Blanche H, Christiansen L, Paca AA, Rea IM, Slagboom E, Flachsbart F, Christensen K, Rimback G, Shrebier S, & Nebel A (2010), No or only population-specific effect of PON1 on human longevity: a comprehensive meta analysis. *Ageing Res Rev*, 9:238–244.

Centers for Disease Control and Prevention (2018), *Physical Activities Guidelines for Americans*. 2nd ed.

Di Lorita C, Long A, Byrne A, Harwood RH, Gladman JRF, Schneider S, Logan P, Bosco AA, & van der Wardt V (2021), Exercise interventions for older adults: a systematic review of meta-analyses. *J Sport Health Sci,* 10:29–47.

Elson L (June 25, 2019), The new exercise guidelines: any changes for you? *Harvard Health Blog.* https://www.health.harvard.edu/blog/the-new-exercise-guidelines-any-changes-for-you-2018121415623

Harb S, Cremer PC, Wu Y, Xu B, Cho L, Menon V, & Jaber WA (2019), Estimated age based on exercise stress testing performance outperforms chronological age in predicting mortality. *Eur J Prev Cardiol,* 10:1177.

Kruger J, Carlson MS, & Buchner D (2007), How active are older Americans? *Prev Chronic Dis,* 4:53–60.

Ludwig MA, Sciamanna CN, Auer BJ, & Argans JP (2021), When American adults move, how do they do so? Trends in physical activity intensity, type, and modality. *J Phys Act Health,* 18:1181–1198.

Reimers CD, Knapp G, & Reimers AK (2012), Does physical activity increase life expectancy? A review of the literature. *J Aging Res,* 2012:9.

Watts EL (2022), Association of leisure time physical activity types and risks of all-cause cardiovascular and cancer mortality among older adults. *JAMA Netw Open,* 5:e2228510.

Weindruch R (December 1, 2006), Caloric Restriction and Aging. *Scientific American.*

Chapter 3: Use Your Brain

Chen LY, Rex CS, Sanaiha Y, Lynch G, & Gall CM (2010), Learning induces neurotrophin signaling at hippocampal synapses. *Proc Natl Acad Sci U S A,* 107(15):7030–7035.

Goforth A (2021), *Does working longer help you live longer.* https://www.benefitspro.com/2021/05/17/does-working-longer-help-you-live-longer/

Kachan D, Fleming LE, Christ S, Muennig P, Prado G, Tannenbaum SL, Ynag X, Caban-Martinez AJ, & Lee DJ (2015), Health status of older US workers and nonworkers, National Health Interview Survey, 1997–2011. *Prev Chronic Dis,* 12:150040.

Krell-Roesch J, Vemuri P, Pink A, Roberts RO, Stokin GB, Mielke MM, Knopman DS, Peterson RC, Kremers WK, & Geda YE (2017), Association between mentally stimulating activities in late life and the outcome of incident mild cognitive impairment, with any analysis of the APOEe4 genotype. *JAMA Neurol,* 74:332–338.

Leibfritz W (2002), Retiring later makes sense. *Korea,* 60:68.

McGee JP, & Wegman DH (2004), *Health and Safety Needs of Older Workers*. National Academies Press.

Westerlund H, Vahtera J, Ferrie JE, Singh-Manoux A, Pentti J, Melchior M, Leineweber C, Jokela M, Siegrist J, Goldberg M, Zins M, & Kivimäki M, (2010), Effect of retirement on major chronic conditions and fatigue: French GAZEL occupational cohort study. *BMJ*, 341:c6149. https://doi. org/10.1136/bmj.c6149

Wu C, Odden MC, Fisher GG, & Stawski RS (2016), The association of retirement age with mortality: a population-based longitudinal study among older adults in the USA. *J Epidemiol Community Health*, 70:917–923.

Zullo JM, Drake D, Aron L, O'Hern P, Dhamne SC, Davidsohn N, & An C (2019), Regulation of lifespan by neural excitation and REST. *Nature*, 574, 359–364.

Chapter 4: Socialization

Holt-Lunstad J, Smith TB, Baker M, Harris T, & Stephenson D (2015), Loneliness and social isolation as risk factors for mortality: a meta-analytic review. *Perspect Psychol Sci*, 10(2):227–237.

Panchal N, Kamal R, Cox C, & Garfield R (July 20, 2021), *The implications of COVID-19 for mental health and substance use*. Kaiser Family Foundation Report. https://www.kff.org/coronavirus-covid-19/issue-brief/the-implications-of-covid-19-for-mental-health-and-substance-use/

Seppala E (June 22, 2020), The loneliness epidemic, and what we can do about it. *Psychology Today*. https://ccare.stanford.edu/psychology-today/the-loneliness-epidemic-and-what-we-can-do-about-it/

Chapter 5: Spiritual Life

Alexander CN, Langer EJ, Newman RI, Chandler HM, & Davies JL (1990), Transcendental meditation, mindfulness, and longevity: an experimental study with the elderly. *J Pers Soc Psychol*, 57:950–964.

Benson H, Dusek JA, Sherwood RN, Lam P, Bethea CF, Carpenter W, Levitsky S, Hill PC, Clem DW, Jain MK, Drumel D, Kopecky SL, Mueller PS, Marek D, Rollins S, & Hibberd PL (2006), Study of the therapeutic effects of intercessory prayer (STEP) in cardiac bypass patients: a multicenter randomized trial of uncertainty and certainty of receiving intercessory prayer. *Am Heart J*, 151:934–942.

Bongiorno P (2012), *How come they're happy and i'm not? The complete natural program for healing depression for good*. Conari Press, Berkeley, CA.

Bruce MA, Martins D, Duru K, Beech BM, Sims M, Harawa N, Vargas R, Kerman D, Nicholas SB, Arleen B, & Norris KC (2017), Church attendance, allostatic load and mortality in middle aged adults. *PLoS ONE* 12(5):e0177618. https://doi.org/10.1371/journal.pone.0177618

Buettner D (2008) *The Blue Zones: Lessons for living longer from the people who've lived the longest*. National Geographic, Washington DC.

Damjanovic AK, Yang Y, Glaser R, Kiecolt-Glaser JK, Nguyen H, Laskowshi B, Zou Y, Beversdorf DQ, & Nan-ping W (2007), Accelerated telomere erosion is associated with a declining immune function of caregivers of Alzheimer's disease patients. *J Immun*, 179:4249–4254.

Ducharme J (February 15, 2018), You asked: do religious people live longer? *Time.* https://time.com/5159848/do-religious-people-live-longer/

Epel ES, Merkin SS, Cawthon R, Blackburn EH, Adler NE, Pletcher MJ, & Seeman TE (2009), The rate of leukocyte telomere shortening predicts mortality from cardiovascular disease in elderly men. *Aging* 1(1):81–88.

Friedman HS & Martin LR (2012) *The longevity project: surprising discoveries for health and long life from the Landmark eight-decade study*. Hudson Street Press, Penguin Group, New York, NY.

Hazen M (2015), *Yoga for longevity*. https://thewholeu.uw.edu/2015/09/28/yoga-for-longevity/

Helm HM, Hays JC, Flint EP, Koenig HG, & Blazer DG (2000), Does private religious activity prolong survival? A six-year follow-up study of 3,851 older adults. *J Gerontology*, 55:400–405.

Herskind AM, McGue M, Holm NV, Sørensen TI, Harvald B, & Vaupel JW (1996) The heritability of human longevity: A population-based study of 2872 Danish twin pairs born 1870-1900. *Hum Genet*, 97(3):319–23. https://doi.org/10.1007/BF02185763

Hoge EA, Chen MM, Orr E, Metcalf CA, Fischer LE, Pollack MH, DeVivo I, & Simon NM (2013), Loving-kindness meditation practice associated with longer telomers in women. Brain Behav Immun, 32:159–163.

House JS, Robbins C, & Metsner HL (1982), The association of social relationships and activities with mortality: prospective evidence from the Tecumseh Community Health Study. *Am J Epidemiol*, 116:123–140.

Hummer R, Rogers R, & Ellison NC (1999), Religious involvement and U.S. adult mortality. *Demography*, 36:273–285.

Koenig HG, Hays JC, & Larson DB (1999), Does religious attendance prolong survival? A six-year follow-up study of 3,968 older adults. *J Gerontol Med Sci*, 54:370–377.

Levine GN, Lange RA, Bairey-Morz CN, Davidson RJ, Jamerson K, Mehta PK, Michos ED, Norris K, Ray IB, Saban KL, Shah T, Stein R, Smith SC, & American Heart Association Council on Clinical Cardiology, Council on Cardiovascular and Stroke Nursing and Council on Hypertension (2017),

Lindqvist D, Epel ES, Mellon SH, Penninx BW, Revesz D, Verhoeven JE, Reus, VI, Lin J, Mahan L, Hough CM, Rosser R, Bersani FS, Blackburn EH, & Wolkowitz OM (2015), Psychiatric disorders and leukocyte telomer length: underlying mechanisms linking mental illness with cellular aging. *Neurosci Behav Rev.* 55L:333–364.

Meditation and cardiovascular risk reduction, a scientific statement from the American Heart Association. *J Amer Heart Assoc*, 10:1061.

Mendioroz M, Puebla-Guedea M, & Montero-Marin J (2020) Telomere length correlates with subtelomeric DNA methylation in long-term mindfulness practitioners. *Scientific Rep.* 10:4564.

Oman D, & Reed D (1998), Religion and mortality among the community-dwelling elderly. *Am J Public Health*, 88:1469–1475.

Ramban, Deuteronomy 22:6–7. https://www.bible.com/bible/compare/DEU.22.6

Shanshan LJ, Sampfer MJ, Williams DR, & VanderWeele Tj (2016), Association of religious service attendance with mortality among women. *JAMA Inten Med*, 176:777–785.

Simon NM, Smoller JW, McNamara KL, Maser RS, Zalta AK, Pollack MH, Nierenberg AA, Fava M, & Wong KK (2006) Telomere shortening and mood disorders: preliminary support for a chronic stress model of accelerated aging. *Biol Psychiatry*, 60(5):432–5.

Strawbridge WJ, Choen RD, Hema SJ, & Kaplan GA (1997), Frequent attendance at religious services and mortality over 28 years. *Am J Public Health*, 87:957–961.

Thorpe M, & Link R (2020), 12 science-based benefits of meditation. Healthline, www.healthline.com/nutrition/12-benefits-of-meditation

Tolahunase M, Sagar R, & Dads R (2017), Impact of yoga and meditation on cellular aging in apparently healthy individuals: a prospective, open-label single-arm exploratory study. *Oxid Med Cell Longev*, 2017:7928981.

Vakonaki E, Tsiminikaki T, Plaitis S, Fragkiadaki P, Tsoukalas D, Katsikantami I, Vaki G, Tzatzaraki MN, Spandidos DA, & Tsatsakis AM

(2018) Common mental disorders and association with telomere length. *Biomed Rep*, 8(2):111–116.

Zuckerman DM, Kast SV, & Ostfeld AM (1984), Psychosocial predictors of mortality among the elderly poor. *Am J Epidemiol*, 119:410–423.

Chapter 6: Keep Having Sex

Abdollahi H, Mollahosseini A, Lane JT, & Mohammad M (2017), A pilot study on using an intelligent life-like robot as a companion for elderly individuals with dementia and depression. *2017 IEEE-RAS 17th International Conference on Humanoid Robotics (Humanoids)*, Birmingham:541–546.

Adaikan PG (2014), Can sexual health contribute to longevity? *Transl Androl Urol*, 3:10.

Castleman M (2017), The prescription for a longer life? More sex. *Psychology Today*, https://www.psychologytoday.com/us/blog/all-about-sex/201705/the-prescription-longer-life-more-sex

Davey-Smith GD, Frankel S, & Yarnell J (1997), Sex and death: are they related? Findings from the Caerphilly cohort study. *BMJ*, 315:1641.

De Baca TC, Epel ES, Robies TF, Coccia M, Gilbert, Puterman E, & Prather AA (2017), Sexual intimacy in couples is associated with longer telomere length. *Psychoneuroendocrinology*, 81:46–51.

Hodis HN, Mack WJ, Henderson VW, Shoupe D, Budoff MJ, Hwang-Levine J, Li Y, Feng M, Dustin L, Kono N, Stanczyk FZ, Selzer RH, Azen SP & the ELITE Research Group (2016), Vascular effects of early versus late postmenopausal treatment with estradiol. *N Engl J Med*, 374:1221–1231.

Kuzmarov IW, & Bain J (2009), Sexuality in the aging couple, Part II: the aging male. *Geriatr Aging*, 12:53–57.

Lindau ST, & Gavrilova N (2010), Sex, health, and years of sexually active life gained due to good health: evidence from two US population based cross sectional surveys of ageing. *BMJ*, 340:810.

Maras M, & Shapiro LR (2017), Child sex dolls and robots: more than just an uncanny valley. *J Internet Law*, 21:3–21.

Masters WH, & Johnson VE (1970), *Human Sexual Inadequacy*. Boston Little Brown.

Paganini-Hill A, Corrada MM, & Kawas CH (2018), Increased longevity in older users of postmenopausal estrogen therapy: the Leisure World Cohort Study. *Metabolism*, 25:1256–1261.

Persson G (1981), Five-year mortality in a 70-year-old population in relation to psychiatric diagnosis, personality, sexuality, and early parental death. *Acta Psychiatr Scand*, 64:244.

Stanworth RD & Jones TH (2008) Testosterone for the aging male; current evidence and recommended practice. *Clin Interv Aging*. 3(1):25–44.

Warner J (2010), Good health boosts social life expectancy. WebMD, https://www.linkedin.com/posts/joncwarner_the-regional-geography-of-us-life-expectancy-activity-7114594854730399744-x8Xq/

Chapter 7: Role of the Microbiome in Health

Blaser MJ (2016), Antibiotic use and its consequences for the normal microbiome. *Science,* 352:544–545.

Brandt LJ (2012), Fecal transplantation for the treatment of *Clostridium difficile infection, Gastroenterol Hepatol (NY)*, 8:191–194.

Cai T, Ye X, Yong H, Song B, Zheng X, Cui B, Zhang F, Lu Y, Miao, H., & Ding D (2018), Fecal microbiota transplantation relieve painful diabetic neuropathy. *Medicine (Baltimore),* 97:e13543.

Carpenter S (2012), That gut feeling. *Amer Psych Assoc Monitor*, 43:50–55.

Clemente JC, Ursell LK, Parfrey LW, & Knigh R (2012), The impact of the gut microbiota on human health: an integrative view. Cell, 148(6):1258–1270.

Grenham S, Clarke G, Cryan JF, & Dinan TG (2011), Brain–gut–microbe communication in health and disease. Front Physiol, 2:94–106.

Gutin L, Piceno Y, Fadrosh D, Lynch K, Zydek M, Kassam Z, LaMere B, Terdiman J, Averil MA, Somsouk M, Lynch S, & Najwa El-Nachef N (2019), Fecal microbiota transplant for Crohn's disease: a study evaluating safety, efficacy, and microbiome profile. *United European Gastroenterol J,* 7:807–814.

Harvard T.H. Chan School of Public Health (2023), *The Nutrition Source: The Microbiome.* https://health.harvard,edu/nutritionsource/microbiome

Harvard Health Publishing (2021) *Diet, disease, and the microbiome,* https://www.health.harvard.edu/blog/diet-disease-and-the-microbiome-2021042122400

Hassouneh R, & Bajaj JS (2021), Gut microbiota modulation and fecal transplantation: an overview on innovative strategies for hepatic encephalopathy treatment. *J Clin Med*, 10:330–342.

Jameson KG, Olson CA, Kazmi SA, & Hsiao EY (2020), Toward understanding microbiome-neuronal signaling. *Mol Cell*, 21:577–583.

Karmakar S, & Lal G (2021), Role of serotonin receptor signaling in cancer cells and anti-tumor immunity. Theranostics, 11:5296–5312.

Kohn D (2015), When gut bacteria change brain function. *Atlantic*, Retrieved June 24, 2015.

Lee KH, Song Y, Wu W, Yu K, & Zhang G (2020), The gut microbiota, environmental factors, and links to the development of food allergy. *Clin Mol Allergy*, 10:1186.

Lopetuso LR, Ianiro G, Allegretti JR, Bibbo S, Gasbarrini A, Scaldaferri F, & Cammarota G (2020), Fecal transplantation for ulcerative colitis: current evidence and future applications. *Expert Opin Biol Ther*, 20:343–351.

Makkawi S, Camara-Lemarroy C, & Metz L (2018), Fecal microbiota transplantation associated with 10 years of stability in a patient with secondary progressive multiple sclerosis. *Neurol Neuroimmunol Neuroinflamm*, 5:459–462.

Meyyappan AC, Forth E, Wallace CJK, & Miley R (2020), Effect of fecal microbiota transplant on symptoms of psychiatric disorders: a systemic review. *BMC Psychiatry*, 20:299–305.

Mossner R, Daniel S, Schmitt A, Albert D, & Lesch KP (2001), Modulation of serotonin transporter function by interleukin-4. *Life Sciences*, 68:873–880.

Napolitano M, & Covasa M (2020), Microbiota transplant in the treatment of obesity and diabetes: current and future perspectives. *Front Microbiol*, 11:590370.

Sender R, Fuchs S, & Milo R (2016), Revised estimates for the number of human and bacteria cell in the body. *PLoS Biol*, 10:1371–1385.3

Terry N, & Margolis KG (2017), Serotonergic mechanisms regulating the GI tract: experimental evidence and therapeutic relevance. Handb Exp Pharmacol, 239:319–342.

Tomova A, Bukovsky I, Rembert E, Yonas W, Alwarith J, Barnard ND, & Kahleova H (2019), The effects of vegetarian and vegan diets on Gut Microbiota. *Front Nutr*, 6:6–16.

Chapter 8: Can Stem Cells Help?

Bellantuono I (2018), Find drugs that delay many diseases of old age. *Nature*, https://www.nature.com/articles/d41586-018-01668-0

Rožman P (2019), How could we slow or reverse the human aging process and extend the healthy life span with heterochronous autologous hematopoietic stem cell transplantation. *Rejuvenation Res,* 23:159–170. https://www.ncbi.nlm.nih.gov/pubmed/31203790

Turner L, & Knoepfler P (2016), Selling stem cells in the USA: assessing the direct to consumer industry. *Cell Stem Cell*, 19:154–157.

Ullah M, & Sun Z (2018), Stem cells and anti-aging genes: double-edged sword—do the same job of life extension. *Stem Cell Res Ther*, 9. https://stemcellres.biomedcentral.com/articles/10.1186/s13287-017-0746-4

Zhang Y, Kim MS, Jia B, Yan J, Zuniga-Hertz JP, Han C, & Cai DS (2017), Hypothalamic stem cells control ageing speed partly through exosomal miRNAs. *Nature,* 548:52–57.

Chapter 10: Traditional and Complementary Medicine

Brody JE (2016), Air pollution takes an invisible tell on health. *New York Times*, November 14, 2016.

Cockle SM, Haller J, Simber S, & Dawe RA (2000), The influence of multivitamins on cognitive function and mood in the elderly. *Aging Ment Health*, 4(4):339–353.

DeSai K, Huang DO, Lakhandwala A, Fernandez A, Riaz IB, & Alpert J (2014), The role of vitamin supplementation on the prevention of cardiovascular disease events. *Clin Cardiol*, 37:576–581.

Gualiare E, Stranges S, Murrow C, Appel W, & Miller ER (2013), Enough is enough: stop wasting money on vitamin and mineral supplements. *Ann Intern Med,* 159:850–851.

Johns Hopkins Medicine (2021), *Types of complementary and alternative medicine*. https://www.hopkinsmedicine.org/health/wellness-and-prevention/types-of-complementary-and-alternative-medicine

Kantor ED, Rehn CD, Du M, White E, & Giovanni EL (2016), Trends in dietary supplement use among U.S. adults from 1996–2012. *JAMA*, 316:1464–1474.

Phutrakool P, & Pongpirul K (2022), Acceptance and use of complementary and alternative medicine among medical specialists: a 15-year systematic review and data synthesis. *Syst Rev,* 11:10.

Chapter 11: How and When to Retire

Levy EG, & Spiro E (2022), *Investing 101 for Physicians: How to Invest Wisely and Sleep Well at Night*. Levy Press, Miami, FL

Chapter 12: Inflammation

Chu AJ (2011), Tissue factor, blood coagulation, and beyond: an overview. *Int J Inflam*, 2011:367284.

Chung HY, Kim DH, Lee EK, Chung KW, Chung S, Lee B, Seo AY, Chung JH, Jung YS, Im E, Lee J, Kim ND, Choi YJ, Im DS, & Yu BP (2019), Redefining chronic inflammation in aging and age-related diseases: proposal of the senoinflammation concept. *Aging Dis*, 1(2):367–382.

Claesson MJ, Jeffery IB, Conde S, Power SE, O'Connor EM, & Cusack S (2011), Gut microbiota composition correlates with diet and health in the elderly. *Nature*, 488(7410):178–184.

Freund A, Orjalo AV, Desprez PY, & Campisi I (2010), Inflammatory networks during cellular senescence: causes and consequences. *Trends Mol Med*, 16(5):238–246.

Jeon OH, Kim C, Laberge RM, Demaria M, Rathod S, & Vasserot AP (2017), Local clearance of senescent cells attenuates the development of post-traumatic osteoarthritis and creates a pro-regenerative environment. *Nat Med*, 23(6):775–781.

Nicklas BJ, Hsu FC, Brinkley TJ, Church T, Goodpaster BH, Kritchevsky SB, & Pahor M (2008), Exercise training and plasma C-reactive protein and interleukin-6 in elderly people. *J Amer Geriatr Soc*, 56(11):2045–2052.

Pottratz ST, & Bellido T (1994), 17-beta estradiol inhibits expression of human interleukin-6 promoter-report constructs by a receptor-dependent mechanism. *J Clin Invest*, 93(3):944–950.

Sanada F, Tariyama Y, Muratsu J, Ofsu R, Shimizu H, Rakugi H, & Morishita R (2018), Source of chronic inflammation in aging. *Front Cardiovasc Med*, 5:12–17.

Singh T, & Newman AB (2011), Inflammatory markers in population studies of aging. *Ageing Res Rev*, 10(3):319–329.

Sparkenbaugh EM, Chantrahammachart P, Mickelson J, van Ryn J, Hebbel RP, & Monroe DM (2014), Differential contribution of FXa and thrombin to vascular inflammation in a mouse model of sickle cell disease. *Blood*, 123(11):1747–1756.

Zhang Q, Raoof M, Chey Y, Sumi Y, Sursal T, & Junger W (2010), Circulating mitochondrial DAMPs cause inflammatory responses to injury. *Nature*, 464:104–107.

Chapter 13: For the Future

Anisimov V (2013), Metformin: do we finally have an anti-aging drug? *Cell Cycle*, 126:3483–3489.

Blagosklonny MV (2019), Rapamycin for longevity: opinion article. *Aging*, 11:19.

Childs BG, Durik M, Baker DJ, & van Deursen JM (2015), Aging and longevity in the simplest animals and the quest for immortality. *Ageing Res Rev*, 16:66–82.

Fang Y, Doyle MF, Chen J, Alosco ML, Mez J, Satizabel CL, Qui WQ, Murabilto JM, & Lunetta KL (2022), Association between inflammatory biomarkers and cognitive aging. *PLoS One*, 17(9):e0274350.https://doi.org/10.1371/journal.pone.0274350

Foley KE (November 5, 2017), A startup that charges $8,000 for young blood transfusions swears they're worth every penny. *Quartz*.

Fontana L, Partridge L, & Longo VD (2010), Extending healthy life span—from yeast to humans. *Science*, 328:321–326.

Graziotto J, Cao K, Collins F, & Krainc D (2012), Rapamycin activates autophagy in Hutchinson-Gilford progeria syndrome. *Autophagy*, 8(1):147–151.

Harrison D, Strong R, Sharp Z, Nelson JF, Astle CM, Flurkey K, Nadon NL, Wilkinson JE, Frenkel K, Carter CS, Pahor M, Javors MA, Fernandez E, & Miller RA (2009), Rapamycin fed late in life extends lifespan in genetically heterogeneous mice. *Nature*, 460(7253):392–395.

Hughes J (October 20, 2011), Transhumanism. In: Bainbridge W, ed. *Leadership in Science and Technology: A Reference Handbook*. Sage Publications:p. 587.

Life Extension (2023), Wikipedia. https://en.wikipedia.org/wiki/Life_extension.

Japsen B (July 17, 2009), AMA report questions science behind using hormones as anti-aging treatment. *The Chicago Tribune*. http://articles.chicagotribune.com/2009-06-15/news/0906140132_1_ anti-aging-hormones-ama-council

Kaeberlein M (2010), Resveratrol and rapamycin: are they anti=aging drugs? *BioEssays*, 32:96–99.

Karasek M (2004), Melatonin, human aging, and age-related diseases. *Exp Gerontol*, 35:1723–1729.

Kim BK, & Park SK (2020), Phosphatidylserine modulates response to oxidative stress through hormesis and increases life span via DAF-12 in *Caenorhabditis elegans*. *Biogerontology*, 21:231–244.

Kirkland J, & Tchkonia T (2015), Clinical strategies and animal models for developing senolytic agents. *Exp Gerontol*, 68:19–25.

Kirkland J & Zhu Y (2022), *Senolytic drugs boost key protective protein*. https://mcpress.mayoclinic.org/research-innovation/senolytic-drugs-boost-key-protective-protein/

Knoll J (1988), Extension of life span of rats by long-term (-)deprenyl treatment. *Mt Sinai J Med*, 55:67–74.

Kraus WE, Bhapkar M, Huffman KM, Pieper CF, Das SK, Redman LM, Villareal DT, Rochon J, Roberts SB, Ravujssin E, Holloszy JO, & Fontana LF (2019), Two years of calorie restriction and cardiometabolic rate (CALERIE): exploratory outcomes of a multicenter, phase 2, randomized control trial. *Lancet*, 7:673–683.

Lamming D, Ye L, Sabatini D, & Baur J (2013), Rapalogs and mTOR inhibitors as anti-aging therapeutics. *J Clin Invest,* 123(3):980–989.

Lifeboatfoundation (2002), *William Faloon*. https://lifeboat.com/ex/bios. william.faloon

Martel J, Ojcius DM, Wu CY, Peng HH, Voisin L, & Perfettini JL (2020), Emerging use of senolytics and senomorphics against aging and chronic diseases. *Med Res Rev*, 40:2114–2131.

Maxmen A (November 5, 2017), Questionable "young blood" transfusions offered in U.S. as anti-aging remedy. *MIT Technology Review*. https://cdn.technologyreview.com/s/603242/questionable-young-blood-transfusions-offered-in-us-as-anti-aging-remedy/

McCormack D, & McFadden D (2013), A review of pterostilbene antioxidant activity and disease modification. *Oxid Med Cell Longev*, 2013:575482. https://pubmed.ncbi.nlm.nih.gov

McDonald RB & Ramsey JJ (2010), Honoring Clive McCay and 75 years of caloric restriction research. *J Nutr.* 140(7):1205–1210.

Olshansky SJ, Hayflick L, & Carnes BA (2002), Position statement on human aging. *J Gerontol*, 57:292–297.

Ostfeld A, Smith CM, & Stotsky BA (1977), The systemic use of procaine in the treatment of the elderly: a review. *J Am Geriatr Soc*, 25:1–19.

Perls T (2013), The reappearance of procaine hydrochloride (Gerovital H3) for antiaging. *J Am Geriatr Soc*, 61:1024–1025.

Ruehl WW, Entriken TL, Muggenburg BA, Bruvette DS, Griffith WC, & Hanh FF (1997), Treatment with L-deprenyl prolongs life in elderly dogs. *Life Sci*, 61a:1037–1044.

Samaras N, Samaras D, Frangos E, Forster A, & Philippe J (2013), A review of age-related Dehydroepiandrosterone decline and its association with well-known geriatric syndromes: is treatment beneficial? *Rejuvenation Res*, 16:285–294.

Sattler FR (2013), Growth hormone in the aging male. *Best Pract Res ClinEndocrinol Metab*, 27:541–555.

Sobh R, & Martin BA (2011), Feedback information and consumer motivation. The moderating role of positive and negative reference values in self-regulation. *Eur J Mark,* 45:963–986.

Statista (2022), Statista Research Department, https://www.statista.com/statistics/509679/value-of-the-global-anti-aging-market/

Tee AR (2018), The Target of rapamycin and mechanisms of cell growth. *Int J Mol Sci,* 19(3):880.

Wikipedia, *Live extension.* https://en.wikipedia.org/wiki/Live_extension

Wei M, Brandhaorst S, Shelehich M, Mirzael H, Cheng CW, Budnick A, Groten S, Mack WJ, Guen E, & Lungo V (2017), Fasting-mimicking diet and markers/risk factors for aging, diabetes, cancer, and cardiovascular disease. *Sci Transl Med,* 9:377.

Zhu Y, Prata LGPL, Gerdes EOW, Netto JME, Pirtskhalava T, Giorgadze N, Tripathi U, Inman CL, Johnson KO, Xue A, Palmer AK, Chen T, Schaefer K, Justice JN, Nambiar AM, Musi N, Kritchevsky SB, Chen J, Khosta S, Jurk D, Schafer MJ, Tchkonia T, & Kirland JL (2022), Orally-active, clinically-translatable senolytics restore α-Klotho in mice and humans. *eBioMedicine* 2022;77:103912. https://doi.org/10.1016/j.ebiom.2022.103912

Appendix A: Going Out to Dinner

Burke L (2017), Eating out may be too much of a temptation for dieters. *American Heart Association News,* https://news.heart.org/eating-out-may-be-too-much-of-a-temptation-for-dieters/

Urban LE, Weber JL, Heyman MD, Schmidt RL, Verstraete S, Lowery NS, Das SR, Schleicher MN, Rogers G, Economo SC, Masters WA, & Roberts SB (2016), Energy contents of frequently ordered restaurant meals and comparison with human energy requirements and U.S. Department of Agriculture database information: a multisite randomized study. *J Acad Nutr Diet,* 116:590–598.

Appendix C: Too Good to Be True

Bartke A (2019), Growth hormone and aging: updated review. *World J Mens Health,* 37:19–30.

Vitale G, Pellegrino G, Vollery M, & Hofland LJ (2019), Role of IGF-1 system in the modulation of longevity: controversies and new insights from a centenarian's perspective. *Pront Endocrinol (Lausanne),* 10:27–52.

Index

7-Eleven, 231
16:8, 31

Abdollahi H, 93
absolute intensity, exercise, 50
acetylation, 153
Acetyl-L-carnitine (ALC), 158–159
"acrylamide", 11
acute inflammation, 141
Adaikan PG, 93
adult stem cells, 105
aerobic activity, 49–50
agave, 27
age management, 241
aging
    contributing factors toward, 109
    stem cells role in, 107–109
air-popped popcorn, 14–15
Airport food options, Miami International
    Airport, 203
air travels, food consumption during, 38
alcohol consumption, 27, 29
allogenic culture, 112
Alzheimer's disease, 105
Amazon Prime, 16
American and ethnic restaurants
    Miami, FL, 177
    types of, 175
American Association of Retired People
    (AARP), 83, 140
Amyotrophic Lateral Sclerosis (ALS), 105
"anaerobic" bacteria, 97

angiotensin-converting enzyme (ACE)
    inhibitors, 168
animal products, disadvantages, 18–20
Anisimov, Vladimir, 166
anti-aging therapy, 237
Anti-Longevity Mindset, 150
apolipoprotein B (ApoB), 45
aptamer-based proteomics, 152
Argentinian restaurant, Normandy Isle,
    FL, 178
arthritis, 20, 51
artificial sweeteners, 27
Aslan, Ana, 156
Aspen Idea Health program, 70
The Atkins diet, 5, 19
avanafil (Stendia), 92
avocado oil, 13

Baby Boomers, viii, 47
    minimal total activity for, 50–51
bacterio therapy, 98
bad cholesterol levels (LDL), 32
Bain J, 91
balance activities, 53–59
    heart rate monitoring, 56
    indoor activities, 56–57
    intense exercise and longevity, 58
    joining gym, 55
    partnering in, 56
    starting stage, 54, 58
    switching events from time to
        time, 57

Barbecue restaurant, Kansas City, MO, 179

Bartke A, 242

Basal Metabolic Rate (BMR), 161

Beverly Hills Diet, 5

Bezos, Jeff, 150

Bhagavad Gita, 78

bhakti (devotion), 78

biodynamic food, 9

biologics, 148

biomarkers, 152

   for aging, 152

   aptamer-based proteomics, 152

   Botechne, 152

   Epigenetic Testing Kit, 152

   SomaScan, 152

   SpectraCell, 152

   TruAge Complete Collection, 152

Black, Indigenous, and People of Color (BIPOC), 66

Blagosklonny MV, 167–168

Blood-type diet, 5

Blue Zone Dwellers: Lessons for Living Longer from the People Who've Lived the Longest, The, 73

Blue Zones: Lessons for Living Longer from the People Who've Lived the Longest, The, 66

bodywork or touch, 125

bone marrow transplants, 105

Bongiorno P, 73

Botechne, 152

brain imaging study, 68

brain-derived neurotrophic factor (BDNF), 64

brain, using, 60–65

brand selection, 133

Brazilian restaurant, New York City, NY, 180

breakfast, 30–33

   "power breakfast" meeting, 33

   "traditional" breakfast versus intermittent fasting, 33

Buettner D, 66, 73–74

Bulsiewicz, William, 100

Butcherbox, 16

Cacioppo, Stephanie, 67

Calcium, 132

calcium-rich milk, 11

CALERIE (Comprehensive Assessment of Long-term Effects of Reducing Intake of Energy) trial, 161

calories, importance, 10–11

Cambridge Diet, 5

Campbell TC, 40

Campbell TM, 40

Campbell, Colin, 133

cancer, 143

carbonated water11–12, , 25

carbonation, 25

carbon-filtered water, 24

carcinogens (cancer promoters), 11

"cardio" activities, 49

cardiovascular disease, 143

Carpenter S, 97

Carrel, Alexis, 149

casein, in milk, 12–13

casual dining restaurants, healthier choices, 175, 212–232

   Caesar salad, 213

   Edamame, 212

   House salad, 213

   Jasmine rice, 213

   Seasonal vegetables, 213

   Seaweed salad, 212

   Steamed asparagus, 213

   Vegetable roll, 212

Cavinton, 156

celiac disease, 34

cell debris, 144–145

cell senescence (aging), 145–146

centenarians, 2

centrophenoxine, 157

Cheesecake Factory, healthier
     choices, 214

     Caesar salad (without cheese or
          anchovies), 214

     Impossible burger, 214

     Thai lettuce wraps with avocado, 214

     Tossed green salad, 214

Chen LY, 64

chick-burgers, 20

Chinese restaurant San Francisco,
     CA, 181

cholesterol, 161

Choline, 14

Chousalkar K, 14

chronic anemia, 143

chronic inflammation, 141

Chuck E. Cheese, 215

Clean Fifteen, 35–36

Clemente JC, 97

Clostridial colitis, 99–100

Clostridium difficile infection, 99

coagulation, 146

cobalamin, ways to get, 38

cofactors, 131–132

Cohen, Pieter A., 130

complementary medicine, 124–134

concierge medicine, 120

conscientiousness, 76

Continental restaurant, Atlanta, GA, 182

convenience store takeouts, 176

cooked and uncooked diet,
          recommended percentage, 36–37

cooking food, disadvantages, 15

cooking water, 22–26

correction, 137

cosmeceuticals, 114

Cracker Barrel, 214

C-reactive protein, 161

Creutzfeldt-Jakob disease, 154

Cuban restaurant, Tampa, FL, 183

cysteine-rich type 1 protein (CD 163), 152

Davis, Adelle, 30

DeBoer MD, 13

degenerative joint disease, 51

dehydroepiandrosterone (DHEA), 155

deionized water, 23

Delicatessen restaurant, New York City,
     NY, 184

Denny's, 217

     Sauteed vegetable blend, 217

     Steamed rice, 217

     Sweet corn, 217

deprenyl, 158

DeSoto L, 30

dhyana (concentration), 78

diabetes, 143

diet and herbs, 125

diet-drinks, 12

diet soda, 11–12

dimethylaminoethanol (DMAE), 157

direct care, 120

Dirty Dozen, 35–36

distilled water, 23

docosahexaenoic acid (DHA), 19

docosapentaenoic acid (DPA), 19

drinking water, 22–26

Drug Coverage, 116

dysbiosis, 96, 98

eating sugar, 27

E. coli, 14

edamame, 20–21

eggs, 14

Egyptian restaurant, Houston, TX, 185

eicosapentaenoic acid (EPA), 19

electromagnetic therapy, 126

electronic health record (EHR), 121

Ellison, Larry, 150

Elson, Lauren, 46

embryonic stem cells, 105

"endurance", 49

Environmental Working Group (EWG), 16

Epel ES, 73, 89

epigenetic clocks, 153
Epigenetic Testing Kit, 152
equities, 137
erectile dysfunction, 91
estradiol, 87
estrogen, 86, 89
Ethiopian restaurant,
        Washington, D.C., 186
exercise, 44–59. *See also* balance
        activities
    absolute intensity in, 50
    aerobic activity, 49–50
    Baby Boomers, minimal total activity
        for, 50–51
    benefits of, 44–45
    flexibility (stretching), 51–52
    for older adults, guidelines, 48
    intense, 50
    muscle-strengthening activities,
        52–53
    perceived level of intensity, 51
    relative intensity, 50
    weight-bearing exercising, 45
external energy treatments, 126

fad diet, 4
"fake" burgers, 20
fast food restaurants, healthier choices
        at, 175, 206–211
    Acai primo bowl, 208
    Banana, 210
    Beyond burger, 206
    Build your own salad, 207
    Caribbean passion smoothie, 208
    Chunky strawberry bowl, 208
    Corn on the cob, 207
    Corn, 208–209
    Electric berry lemonade
        smoothie, 208
    Go getter (plant based, veggies
        and fruit) smoothie, 208
    Green beans, 208
    Impossible sausage sandwich, 208
    Impossible whopper, 206
    Market salad, 207
    Oatmeal with soymilk, 208
    Quesadilla, 207
    Red beans and rice, 209
    Rice, 28
    Salad, 207
    Side salad, 207
    Spicy Southwest salad, 207
    Summer blackberry smoothie, 208
    Vegan beyond burger, 206
    Veggie, 208
    VegiFi burger (from quinoa), 206
fasting-mimicking diets, 161
fat in milk, 12–13
fecal microbial transplant, 98
fibrinolysis system, 146
filtered water, 23
fisetin, 170
fish as food, 26
Fit for Life, 5
flavonoids, 170
flight travel, food consumption
        during, 38
fluorosis, 25
follow-up tests, 133
food combining concept, 40–41
"Fountain of Youth", 113
French restaurant, Paris, France, 187
fresh "nonorganic" vegetables, 16
Friedman HS, 76
frozen items, 20
frozen vegetables, 16–17
"Full Retirement", 60
future, looking at, 149–172
    aging-associated diseases, 160
    Metformin, 164, 166
    NAD+, 164–165
    Rapamycin, 164, 167
    senolytics and pro-longevity drugs,
        162–163

senomorphic medications and
    pro-longevity medications,
    163–168
very low-calorie diets, 160–162

Gavrilova N, 84
genetically modified organism (GMO),
    20–21, 98
GH3 (Gerovital), 156
"ghrelin" hormone, 5
gluten
    gluten ataxia, 34
    "gluten-free" foods, 33–35
    harms of, 34
Goforth A, 63
going out to dinner, 173–232. See also
    individual restaurants
Graves' disease, 141
Greek restaurant, Chicago, IL, 188
Grenham S, 97
growth hormone, 242
growth hormone–releasing peptide
    (GHRP), 242
gut dysbiosis, 145
gut healing, 242

Hamblin J, 18
Hamburger restaurant, Omaha,
    NE, 189
Hard Rock Café, 218
Hazen, Mary, 79
healthy diet
    social life and, 28–29
healthy eating, 1–43
    calories, importance, 10–11
    plant–based food, 1, 9
    questions and answers 8–43
    voluntarily changing diet, 4
herbs, 125
Hodis HN, 90
Hoge EA, 81
Holt-Lunstad J, 2, 67

homeopathic and oriental practices,
    124–125
honey, 27
Hospital Insurance, 116
Houston's, 219
How Come They're Happy and I'm Not?
    The Complete Natural Program
    for Healing Depression
    for Good, 73
Human Growth Hormone (HGH), 154
Hutchinson-Gilford Progeria
    Syndrome, 167

IHOP, 220
Ikaria, Greece, spiritual life in, 74
immunosenescence, 146
Imperfect Foods, 16
Indian restaurant, Las Vegas, NV, 190
inflammation, 141–148
    acute inflammation, 141
    anti-inflammatory foods, 147
    cell debris, 144–145
    cell senescence (aging), 145–146
    chronic inflammation, 141
    coagulation and fibrinolysis
        system, 146
    consequences of, 143–146
    elevating factors, 142–143
    foods that alleviate, 147–148
    gut dysbiosis, 145
    immediate action for, 146–148
    immunosenescence, 146
    other conditions related to 143
insurance, health care and, 115–123
    conveyor belt medicine, 121
    cost, 117
    coverage, 118
    doctor and hospital choice, 117
    Medicare Supplemental Insurance
        (Medigap), 116
    original Medicare and Medicare
        advantage, differences, 116

original medicare, 119
Part A (Hospital Insurance), 116
Part B (Medical Insurance), 116
Part D (Drug Coverage), 116
traditional medicare, 116
interleukin-6 (IL-6), 142
intermittent fasting, 31–32
"traditional" breakfast and, 33
Ipamorelin, 242
irritable bowel syndrome, 95
Israeli restaurant Philadelphia, PA, 191
Italian restaurant Providence, RI, 192
IVF (in vitro fertilization) lab, 106

J Alexander, 221
Jameson KG, 97
Janov, Arthur, 73
Japanese restaurant,
    Los Angeles, CA, 193
jnana (knowledge), 78
Junk Food Diet, 5

Kachan D, 62
Kaeberlein M, 153
Kantor, Elizabeth D., 130
Karasek M, 159
karma (action), 78
Ketogenic (keto) diet, 5
Knoepfler P, 110
Krell-Roesch J, 64
Kruger J, 46
Kuzmarov IW, 91

lactose in milk, 12–13
Lasheras C, 43
lead contamination, 22
Legal Sea Foods, 222
Leibfritz W, 62
"leptin", 5
leukocyte telomere length (LTL), 44, 73
leukocytosis, 15
Levine GN, 81

life expectancy
    in 1970, 61
Lindau ST, 84
Lion Diet, 5
Loeb, Frances Lehman, 78
Loeb, John L., 78
Loma Linda, California, USA, spiritual
    life in, 74
loneliness, coping with, 68–69
Longevity Mindset, 150
*Longevity Project: Surprising
    Discoveries for Health and
    Long Life from the Landmark
    Eight-Decade Study*, 76
longevity
    and sex, 88
    suggestions for, 233
    of women versus men, 89
LongHorn Steakhouse, 223
Loving-Kindness Meditation
    (LKM), 81
"low-fat" diet, 19

Magnesium, 132
magnetic field therapy, 126
maple syrup, 27
Martin LR, 76
Mayo Clinic Diet, 5
McCay, Clive, 160
meclofenoxate, 157
Medical Insurance, 116
Medicare Supplemental Insurance
    (Medigap), 116
meditation, 79
    science-based benefits of, 80
Mediterranean diet, 6
melatonin, 159–160
membership-medicine, 120
Mendioroz M, 81
meta-analysis, 44–45
Metformin, 164, 166
methylation, 153

Mexican restaurant, San Antonio, TX, 194

Michaelsson K, 12

microbiome role in health, 95–103
  "anaerobic" bacteria, 97
  colonized microbial communities, 97
  gut and nervous system, signaling between, 97
  nurturing microbiome, 100
  pathogenetic (disease-causing) bacteria, 96
  prebiotics, 102
  probiotics, 101
  symbiotic relationship, 96

microgreens, importance, 17

microRNAs, 109

microwaved food, 21

microwaved popcorn, 14–15

MILES (Metformin in Longevity Study), 166

milk
  harmful substances in, 12–13

Miller, Richard, 168

mind work, 126

mindfulness training (MF), 80

minerals, 131–132

Misfits Market, 16

Misto Can, 13

mitochondria, 145

"moais", 74

molecular marker, 152

mono diet, 41

monoamine oxidase (MAO) levels, 156

muscle-strengthening activities, 52–53

NAD+, 164–165

National Health Interview Survey data, 62

neurodegenerative problems, 132

The New England Centenarian Study, xiii

Nicoya Peninsula, Costa Rica, spiritual life in, 74

non-celiac gluten sensitivity, 34

nonorganic vegetables/fruits never be eaten, 35–36

oil, 13
  olive oil, 13
  Omega Oleic Acid oil, 132
  Omega-3 oil, 13
  Omega-6 oil, 13
  Omega-9 oil, 13
  pumpkin oil, 13
  safflower oil, 13
  sesame oil, 13
  vegetable oil, 13

Okinawa diet, 6

Okinawa, Japan, spiritual life in, 74

Olive Garden, 224

olive oil, 13

Omega Oleic Acid oil, 132

omega-3 fatty acids, 8

Omega-3 oil, 13

Omega-6 oil, 13

Omega-9 oil, 13

"Optifast", 6

organic food, 9

organic vegetables, 16

original medicare, 119

osteopenia, 143

osteoporosis, 45

Outback Steakhouse, 225

Paganini-Hill A, 90

Paleo (Paleolithic) diet, 5

parachlorophenoxyacetate (PCPA), 157

Parkinson's disease, 105

Pasta Diet, 5

pescatarians, 28

PF Chang China Bistro, 226

phosphatidylserine, 158

phosphodiesterase type 5 inhibitors (PDE-5i's), 92

physical activity (PA), 44. *See also* exercise
  benefits of, 44–45
Piracetam, 154–155
Pizza restaurant, Brooklyn, NY, 195
plant-based diet, 1, 9, 27–28
  defining, 8–9
  list of, 11
  starting time, 42
  time period to, 40
platelet-rich plasma (PRP) therapy, 112, 240–241
polymyalgia rheumatica (PMR), 143
polyphenols, 100
popcorn, 14–15
  air-popped, 14–15
  microwaved, 14–15
potatoes, 26–27
prebiotics, 102
Primal Therapy, 73
Pritikin Diet, 5
probiotics, 101
progeria, 145
pro-longevity medications, 163–168
protease, 33
protein in meal, 38
"Protein Sparing Modified Fat" program, 6
pterostilbene, 170
Public Goods, 16
pumpkin oil, 13
purified water, 23

quercetin, 170

Rapamycin, 164, 167
raw (uncooked) food, 15
rawtarian, 27–28
rawtarians, 28
Red Lobster, 227
regenerative medicine, 237–238
regional enteritis, 143

relative intensity, exercise, 50
Required Minimum Distributions (RMDs), 140
residential program, 42–43
resveratrol, 170
retainer medicine, 120
retirement, 135–140
  assets distribution, 139
  bonds, 139
  income-generating investments, 138
  Required Minimum Distribution (RMD), 140
  retirement funding, 137
  when and how, 135–140
Reverse Osmosis (RO), 23–24
robot companions, 93
Roman, Andy, 72
Rotation Diet, 5
Rožman P, 108
Russian restaurant, Arlington, VA, 196

safflower oil, 13
Salmonella enteritidis, 14
salt consumption, 13–14
Sanada F, 144
Seafood restaurant, Miami Beach, FL, 197
Seasons 52, 228
selegiline, 158
senescence-associated secretory phenotype (SASP), 163
senolytics and pro-longevity drugs, 162–163
senolytics, 113
senomorphic medications and pro-longevity medications, 163–168
Seppala, Emma, 68
Serotonin, 97
sesame oil, 13
sexual life and health, 83–94
  age related changes in men and, 91–92
  benefits of regular sex, 84

estrogen level, 86
longevity and sex, 88
longevity of women versus men,
    89, 92–94
performance anxiety, 91
spontaneous desire versus
    responsive desire, 86–87
testosterone use, 87–88
short-chain fatty acids (SCFA), 96
signature molecule, 152
sildenafil (Viagra), 92, 94
Simon NM, 72
Sinclair, David, 31
sirtuin-activating compounds
    (STACs), 165
sirtuin-activating polyphenols, 170
Sirtuins (Silent Information
    Regulators), 164
Sizzler, 229
social life and healthy diet, 28–29
    entertaining in home, 29
socialization, 66–71
soda, 11–12
SomaScan, 152
South Beach diet, 5
Spanish restaurant, New Orleans, LA, 198
spastic colon (irritable bowel
    syndrome), 95
SpectraCell, 152
spiritual life, 72–82
    belonging, 75
    conscientiousness, 76
    downshifting, 75
    Ikaria, Greece, 74
    Loma Linda, California, USA, 74
    meaningful work and 76
    natural moving, 75
    Nicoya Peninsula, Costa Rica, 74
    Okinawa, Japan, 74
    plant-based diets in, 75
    purpose, 75
    right tribe, 74

strong social networks, 75
    yoga, 78
spring water, 22
sprouts, importance, 17
"Staff of Life", 33
starvation, 31
Steak House restaurant, Chicago, IL, 199
stem cells, 104–114
    adult stem cells, 105
    aging and, 107–109
    allogenic culture, 112
    birth tissues (umbilical cord blood or
        amniotic fluid), 112
    embryonic stem cells, 105
    expenses associated with, 111–112
    in anti-aging, 111
    perinatal stem cells, 105
    platelet-rich plasma (PRP)
        injections, 112
    real stuff of, 109–114
    sources, 105
stimulation of senses, 126
sugar in milk, 12–13
Sun Z, 108
supplements, 131–132
    guide for, 132–133

tadalafil (Cialis), 92
TAME (Targeting Aging with Metformin),
    166
tap water, 22
T cells, 97
telomeres, 80
testosterone use, 87–88
TGI Fridays, 230
Thai restaurant, Toronto, Canada, 200
Thiel, Peter, 150
Thrive Market, 16
Thymosin A1, 242
Thymosin B4 (TB4), 242
tissue healing and repair, 242
tofu, 20–21

Tomova A, 100
trace vitamins, 131–132
traditional and complementary
        medicine, 124–134
    bodywork or touch, 125
    brand selection, 133
    cofactors, 131–132
    diet and herbs, 125
    external energy treatments, 126
    follow-up tests, 133
    homeopathic and oriental practices,
        124–125
    minerals, 131–132
    supplements, 131–132
    trace vitamins, 131–132
transcendental meditation (TM)
        program, 80
triglycerides, 45, 161
trimethylamine N-oxide (MRAO), 14
TruAge Complete Collection, 152
Tucker KL, 12
tumor necrosis factor-α (TNF-α) 142
Turkish restaurant, Dallas, TX, 201
Turner L, 110

ulcerative colitis (UC), 99
Ullah M, 108
ultrafiltered water, 24
ultraviolet oxidized water, 24
uncooked (raw) food, 15

vacation, food consumption during, 37
Vakonaki E, 72
VanderWeele, Tyler J., 78
vardenafil (Levitra), 92
vascular dementia, 58
vegan, 27–28
vegan, but are not healthy foods, 28
"Vegan diets", 8
vegetable oil, 13
vegetables purchase, sources of, 16
vegetarian, 27–28

vegetarian restaurant, New York City,
        NY, 202
veggie-bacon, 20
veggie-sausage, 20
very low-calorie diets, 160–162
Vinpocetine, 156
Vitale G, 242
Vitamin B, 96
Vitamin B12 (cobalamin), 38–40, 96
    deficiency, 39
    ways to get, 38–40
Vitamin B6, 39
Vitamin B9 (folic acid), 39
Vitamin D deficiency, 132
Vitamin K, 96
vitamin water, 12
voluntarily changing our diet always
        happens for a reason, 4

Walker, Allan, 101
water consumption, 22–26
    carbon-filtered water, 24
    deionized water, 23
    distilled water, 23
    drinking water, 22–26
    filtered water, 23
    purified water, 23
    Reverse Osmosis (RO), 23–24
    spring water, 22
    tap water, 22
    ultrafiltered water, 24
    ultraviolet oxidized water, 24
    water used in cooking, 22–26
WaWa, 232
weight loss 4
Westerlund H, 63
What You Should Know about Plant-
        Based Diets—Cleveland Clinic, 40
wheat allergy, 34
Whole Foods buffet, 204
Widower's Syndrome, 91
Wilkinson MJ, 32

Winfrey, Oprah, 6
Wu C, 62

Yoga and Meditation–based lifestyle
     intervention (YMLI), 81
Yoga, 52
Yoga, 78
     bhakti (devotion), 78
     dhyana (concentration), 78

jnana (knowledge), 78
karma (action), 78
types, 78

Zhang Y, 109
Zhi-hui L, 30
zombie cells, 113, 162
Zone Diet, 5
Zullo JM, 65

Life-Style

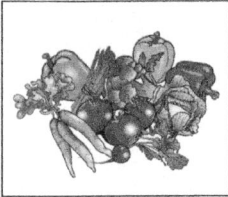

Diet

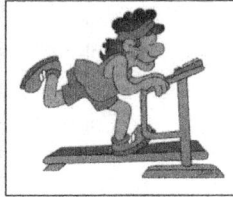

Exercise

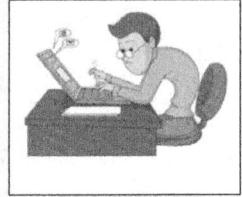

Use your brain

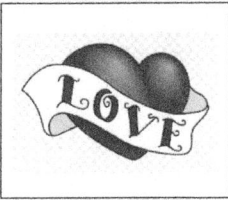

Keep having sex

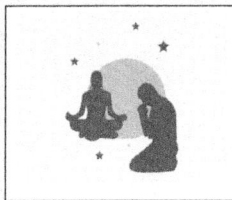

Spirituality

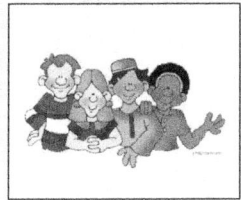

Socialization

+ Biologicals

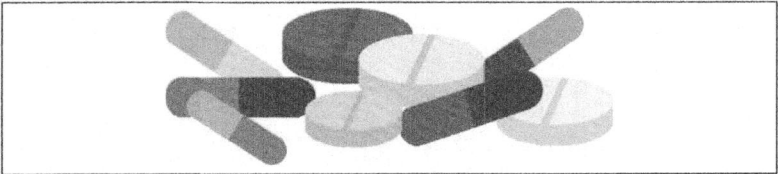

= Live to 120

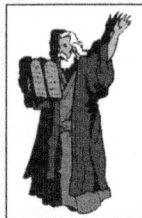

Made in the USA
Coppell, TX
09 April 2025

48098966R00157